# Yoga Therapy for Every Special Child

*of related interest*

**The Healing Power of Mudras**
**The Yoga of the Hands**
*Rajendar Menen*
ISBN 978 1 84819 043 6

**Integrated Yoga**
**Yoga with a Sensory Integrative Approach**
*Nicole Cuomo*
ISBN 978 1 84310 862 7

**Yoga for Children with Autism Spectrum Disorders**
**A Step-by-Step Guide for Parents and Caregivers**
*Dion E. Betts and Stacey W. Betts*
*Forewords by Louise Goldberg, Registered Yoga Teacher and Joshua S. Betts*
ISBN 978 1 84310 817 7

**Curves, Twists and Bends**
**A Practical Guide to Pilates for Scoliosis**
*Annette Wellings with Alan Herdman*
ISBN 978 1 84819 025 2

# Yoga Therapy for Every Special Child

## Meeting Needs in a Natural Setting

Nancy Williams

*Illustrated by Leslie White*

SINGING DRAGON
LONDON AND PHILADELPHIA

First published in 2010
by Singing Dragon
an imprint of Jessica Kingsley Publishers
116 Pentonville Road
London N1 9JB, UK
and
400 Market Street, Suite 400
Philadelphia, PA 19106, USA

*www.singing-dragon.com*

Copyright © Nancy Williams 2010
Illustrations copyright © Leslie White 2010

**Library of Congress Cataloging in Publication Data**
A CIP catalog record for this book is available from the Library of Congress

**British Library Cataloguing in Publication Data**
A CIP catalogue record for this book is available from the British Library

ISBN 978 1 84819 027 6

Printed and bound in the United States by
Thomson-Shore, 7300 W. Joy Road, Dexter, MI 48130

This book is dedicated to the yogis

Alana, Alex, Alexis, Aleyda, Amelia, Amy, Annika, Angelita, Benjamin, Brittany, Casey, Chase, Claire, Dominique, Edgar, Eliza, Elizabeth, Gaylen, Holly, Irene, Jacob, Jenna, Jeremy, Joey, Jonathan, Josh, Katie, Katy, Kelsey, Lia, Liam, Linda, Lon, Luis, Mac, Matthew, Mia, Michael, Nancy, Nicky, Olive, Oliver, Robert, Robin, Russel, Salicia, Selina, Sloane, Steven, Taylor, Tim, Tito, Valerie, Zachary and Zoe.

# ACKNOWLEDGEMENTS

I thank my parents, Phylis and Glen, who were great teachers of love and service. Much gratitude to Kate and Clay for the opportunity to know the joys of parenting. You are my greatest gifts.

Thank you to the parents who believed in yoga therapy and lovingly provided their children the opportunity to learn and grow in an innovative therapy setting.

Gratitude to Priscilla Potter for starting Tucson, Arizona's "The Yoga Connection" and sharing her wisdom in the love of yoga. To the artist, my sister, who devoted so many hours of time to create the essence of the children who have graced my life in yoga therapy, thank you!

Much gratitude to Cynthia, Denise, Marie and Pat for their weekly practice of the yoga program I developed for the children. I thank Tim for providing adult feedback as to how yoga impacts the body of a person living with cerebral palsy.

I express love and thankfulness to my best friend and fiancé, Tom, who has been a strong support for me during the manuscript years.

Most of all, I thank Spirit for guiding me to yoga therapy and to the awareness that life is as spectacular as I am able to imagine and create it!

# CONTENTS

# PREFACE

I wrote this book so that I could share the fundamentals of yoga therapy and some of the wonderful exercises that have evolved out of ten years of teaching therapy to children with special needs. I needed a well organized, comprehensive and engaging tool to offer parents, and those who wish to teach parents, the effective and simple techniques of yoga therapy.

What does yoga therapy look like? It looks like a group of beautiful special needs children learning and using the important components of a gentle Hatha yoga practice to improve each and every aspect of their lives. What are these components? They include (but are not limited to) breath work, sequenced hand postures performed while chanting, a carefully choreographed sequence of gentle yoga poses and the opportunity to integrate all of these skills while relaxing inward to visualize a guided meditation. What do I hope to accomplish with yoga therapy? I hope to help each child visualize their dreams through a practice of inner creation and to optimize the use of their bodies through stretches, coordinated poses and rotation. I hope to see transformations that will allow each child to blossom into their highest potential by improving skills in all areas of development, while amplifying the quality of their lives.

I enjoy my role as a speech pathologist helping shape words from thoughts for so many children. This is the foundation that I created thirty-three years ago, but it is over the last ten, following my certification as a yoga teacher, that everything in my life has become better and brighter—because that is what happens when you bring yoga into your life.

Yoga helped me breathe deeper, twist further, balance better, bend with ease, appreciate myself and others more, while teaching me that I am the responsible creator in my life.

In this book, you will learn how to bring this joy into your child's life, by teaching them the components of a yoga practice.

With the thorough descriptions of each section of the program, accompanying illustrations and a glossary of terms, the yoga program may be easily practiced.

Yoga blessings,

Nancy

# 1

## INTRODUCTION

As precious infant fingers grasp your own, the miracle of physical movement, whether reflexively or with intention, is a beautiful reminder of the body's capabilities from birth. When observing the most basic postures of a baby, it is evident that each level of physical mastery begins with the motivation to move.

### NORMAL DEVELOPMENT

As a baby repeatedly exercises a specific part of its body, the flexion (a folding in and bending of the body) and extension (a lengthening and opening of the body) by the muscles that are used gradually develop the strength to achieve upward movement against gravity. Repeated practice and strengthening of the muscles facilitates the balance that is necessary in order to maintain the base of support for this new physical posture.

The skill of balance in a posture, combined with a baby's curiosity to explore his environment, precipitates movement and subsequent rotation of the body. It is through the balance of flexion, extension and rotation of the body that the spiraling movement upward against gravity is achieved. Within one year of life, we observe a baby transition from back and tummy lying, through several postural transitions and into an upright standing posture, prepared to take the first steps. It is important to remember the many hours of practice that are required for a healthy, uncompromised body and mind to achieve the ability to stand and move forward with a steady gait.

During this important first year of development the core of the body, or torso, is strengthened. This core stability of the body allows the young one to develop more refined movement for the various skills that will be needed to relate to his environment. With the combined experience of exploration and a stronger torso, the body and mind can work as one to provide the toddler success in feeding, explorative play and successful communication.

## DEVELOPMENTAL CHALLENGES

Only through this awareness of unimpeded development can we comprehend the needs and challenges of a body or mind that has been compromised at birth or during subsequent years of life. When the flow of movement and exploration is difficult or hindered in any area of development and compensations are only marginally effective, the total experience for the baby or toddler may not be perceived as rewarding. When expectations of this young one are focused on a desired result that cannot be achieved as expected, frustration and a reduced level of motivation may occur.

The high level of frustration that can be experienced by the special needs child makes it imperative to seek an intervention technique that allows for small steps toward their optimal performance. Accepting the child's present capabilities while also providing a context for improved skills may create an environment of acceptance, ease and continued success. When intervention provides continual positive reinforcement, the baby or child is more likely to comply with the requests being made.

When a child has special needs in any area of development it is important to use a therapy approach that is easily received by that young one.

## SIMILARITIES BETWEEN YOGA AND NEURO-DEVELOPMENTAL THERAPY

A connection that forever altered my work occurred while I was studying towards teacher's certification in Hatha yoga. As I moved my body through the yoga poses I had created for a gentle beginning yoga class, I realized the transitions mirrored the framework of neuro-developmental therapy (NDT). I had been certified in this therapy approach (Bobath 1980) 14 years prior, and the similarities of both practices became clear. NDT was developed to treat children diagnosed with cerebral palsy and supported a balance of flexion (a folding in and bending of the body) with extension (a lengthening and opening of the body). This balance of flexion and extension was also, I realized, the foundation of yoga—both programs requiring movement through each normal developmental posture from back/front lying, sitting, hands-and-knees, and up into standing. Yoga had additional components, however, highly beneficial features that were not a part of NDT—the delicate skill of moving energy throughout the body, incorporating yogic breathing within each pose, and the inclusion of meditation at the closure of the session. For me, this was the enlightening moment where physical/structural met energetic/regeneration.

## YOGA MEETS THERAPY GOALS

Nine years of using yoga for therapeutic intervention revealed that the simple yoga sequence used in each session supported the needs and goals of the children I was treating. I discovered that yoga naturally exercises and stimulates the skills that are traditionally assessed by multidisciplinary tests that include gross and fine motor, speech and language comprehension and production, as well as quality of function. Addressing traditional therapy goals through the practice of yoga became a study of wonderment as each isolated component of a developmental skill revealed itself to me during the yoga sequence. I discovered that yoga encompassed the integral parts of my training as a therapist and offered a beautiful, creative and enjoyable experience for the fulfillment of desired improvement with each child.

# 2

## THE BENEFITS OF YOGA

The benefits of yoga are heralded in many publications for the healing effects that can be achieved through the use of this ancient practice. Yoga, which means "union," is the word used by the Hindu culture to describe the natural flow of body movements while melding structure and energy. Many authors have reported the benefits of a yoga practice for specific populations and diagnoses. Information and training in the support of yoga benefits has flourished in recent years with the inclusion of yoga for autism spectrum disorder (Betts and Betts 2006), Amy Weintraub's focus on *Yoga for Depression* (Weintraub 2004), and improved functioning of children with sensory integration disorder (Cuomo 2007). Balakrishnan (2009) outlines yoga as a treatment for stuttering. For some time yoga has been a popular choice for those who wish to study a viable practice to enlightenment (Kriyananda 1976). Periodical literature reports yoga as beneficial, in at least a complementary role, for multiple sclerosis, cardiopulmonary function, post-traumatic stress disorder—the list goes on and on. Yoga is becoming more visible and viable as an available service in institutions and programs across the world for the myriad benefits it provides.

To compile a complete list of yoga benefits is nearly impossible, but it is true to say that it improves the quality of life in general and inner connection specifically. Most of all I wish to focus on the best known gifts that yoga has been documented to provide, alongside therapeutic specifics, so as to help parents, therapists or students to become better educated about requesting and implementing yoga for special needs.

## THE BREATH

Breathing is an expansive part of a yoga program. By inhaling through the nose, the breath can be guided more deeply and directed more skillfully. Nasal hair filters and mucosa moisten the air that is taken into the body. When breath is coordinated with yoga postures, previously constricted portions of the body can receive increased blood flow and improved oxygenation. The maximal benefit is accomplished by coordinating the breathing pattern with the natural physiological flow of the body. As yoga postures are guided, the cycle of inhalation and exhalation is explained. During elongation and extension of the body a deep inhalation is natural; conversely, flexing the body automatically expels the breath. As a posture is held the breathing continues, deep and even, directing the oxygen into the open and expanding space. A well oxygenated body relaxes and brainwaves may alter, contributing to an overall feeling of well-being. During a state of altered brainwave function, or meditation, the mind/body integrates information more deeply. The benefits of imprinting positive information while a person is in this state have been reported by many psychiatrists who have used hypnosis to reprogram a previous pattern of behavior.

Many children diagnosed with special needs have experienced difficulties breathing because of structural impairment or physiological compromises. Frequently their chosen resting posture does not allow for maximum intake of oxygen. These children often hold their breath when moved out of their habitual postures. Some children have learned to breathe with their head and neck in extension, while other children demonstrate a shallow breathing cycle with the mouth open. Training a deeper and sustained breathing cycle during yoga poses can break through previous patterns that have become a physiological habit.

Bubble blowing provides visual feedback for the child as she observes the bubbles moving further through space, and becoming larger as exhalations are sustained. As the child learns to guide a deeper breath through her nostrils, she also observes the advantages of graded exhalation with improved breath control for bubble blowing. As she engages in this respiration activity she benefits from increased oxygen as it moves through the vascular system.

Children begin to feel the natural flow of breath in relation to their body. A deep inhalation is easier with an open and extended body, and it is natural to expend the breath as the body folds into flexion. With reminders throughout the yoga session of when to breathe, the child may experience the natural rhythm of a smooth cycle of inhalation and exhalation.

## BODY AWARENESS

Through the slow, guided movements of yoga, a child becomes more aware, as the body reveals pain or tightness while bending, stretching and/or rotating through postures. Taking each pose to a comfortable limit and guiding the breath to that spot can encourage relaxation and loosening, and often reduction in pain. Awareness of tight parts of the body is a guide towards greater care and safety with each posture and provides a baseline from which to work. The child is becoming more aware of each portion of his body and how it moves in various directions. With repeated familiar movements in a context of relaxation, the body learns to move more skillfully, demonstrating flowing, graded transitions.

Directionality is repeatedly practiced as the child is instructed to move, first the right and then left side of the body, through poses that have an excursion to the right, left, upward, downward, laterally, or into twist.

With each breath the child can observe how the body changes during the cycle of inhalation and exhalation. Parents ask each child to observe where their body expands and contracts in relation to a deep breath. This practice cues the child into the changes that may occur as they breathe through a constricted area during a yoga pose.

From the functional task of rolling up the yoga mat (bilateral integration) to determining which leg is the "left one" (directionality), the child has a myriad of experiences that teach him to know his body and how it feels as it supports and moves.

## MOTOR PLANNING

As the child follows the preliminary directions in the therapeutic yoga sequence, there are numerous opportunities for him to practice motor planning skills. Motor planning is the ability to successfully execute a sequence of small, coordinated steps to complete a required task. Examples of motor planning include the steps necessary to perform *namasté* by first bringing the hands together, then moving them up and over the heart spot, and finally bowing. Tibetan bells are utilized to cue the beginning of the yoga sequence and to encourage each child to successfully hold the bells in a pincer grasp. The child then rings the bells, and the quality of his ability to grade his movement can be heard in the soft and pleasantly audible ring tone.

Mudras, or hand postures, are an important component in a yoga class. Mudras are intended to be a fluent sequence of arms, wrists and hand movements that create a picture of flow and beauty. In therapeutic yoga, completing mudras is another opportunity to stimulate and encourage gross and fine motor planning skills. It is through the repeated explanation of each detail within a pose and the sequencing of poses that the child begins to plan his motor movements. The familiar and repetitive order of the yoga therapy sequence supports the success of each child to plan their motor movements with skill.

## SPIRIT OF COMMUNICATION

A precedence of respect is set at the beginning of each yoga class. The teacher and children bow to one another with the spoken word, as well as hand posture, for *namasté*. The meaning of *namasté*, "I honor the light in you", is the first and most important aspect of communication dynamics in the yoga class. Respect for one another is lovingly presented and maintained throughout and after the yoga session.

Yoga naturally facilitates communication skills of gesture, and vocal and verbal production. Pre-verbal children have the opportunity to imitate yoga postures, hand gestures and vocal productions. Through simple chant, or mantra, vowel–consonant and consonant–vowel productions are practiced. Mudras provide opportunities for supporting sign language.

The therapeutic yoga sequence is conducted with the instructor guiding the progression, using both visual demonstration and clear verbal instruction. Each move is guided with the appropriate inhalation and exhalation cycles. Attributes of quality, directionality and number are used during explanations. One-, two- and three-step directions are normal in the yoga sequence at a level that is appropriate for the skill of the child.

Yoga games support the opportunity to engage in social/communicative interactions. Activities such as "Yogi Pogi" and "Yogi Says" are popular with the children and enable them to practice careful listening, as well as develop leadership skills by taking turns at teaching their peer group. Bubble blowing for respiration control allows partners to interact and respect turn-taking skills. Encouragement, praise and respect abound in a therapeutic yoga class.

## BEHAVIORAL SELF-REGULATION

One of the first skills to develop in therapeutic yoga is the ability to self-regulate. Frequently the breath becomes the first area of self-regulating, and the child learns to breathe more slowly and deeply when she becomes anxious. Other reports conclude that children will chant the familiar mantras to ease anxiety, and, in some instances, remove themselves from the environment, if at all possible, and do some yoga poses.

To be able to self-regulate your focus, mood or general expression is a crucial skill for developing social skills. Once a child has been able to modulate his performance by using a technique to quiet, focus and calm himself, he is on the way to improving his ability to interact and succeed in society.

## SOCIAL SKILLS

Yoga improves many things in a child's life, and social skill is typically an area where progress is observed. Learning the respect of self is monumental in effectively engaging with another. The ability to take turns, listen, observe body space and initiate kindness are mutual aspects of a yoga class, as well as a successful social interaction.

Enjoying the yoga program with your child can provide you with opportunities to take turns. When blowing bubbles, you honor your child when it is his turn to blow and he repeats this courtesy when you blow the bubbles. This reciprocal interaction is somewhat different from many daily activities where you, as the parent, deliver advice, food, clothing and instructions to your child. Mutual respect is the intention of the yoga therapy program and provides an opportunity for you to engage in social interaction with your child. Sharing this experience with your child at home builds the skills he will need when interacting with others.

A group format can provide children a natural setting for social interaction. Friends and siblings can be invited to join in the program. Mixing children with differing needs can design a setting where one child's social strength can support another child's social weakness. Mixing children of different ages can provide various experiences of nurturing one another or providing a role model.

The respectful and accepting nature of a yoga class have supported new friendships that have been maintained over years. The level of support provided to one another is truly heart opening.

## UNIVERSAL AWARENESS

Yoga is based on unity and the respect of all. The yoga greeting "*namasté*" sets a precedent of honoring all people, and the child in yoga begins to treat others as he would like to be treated. Harmonizing with chants until two voices become one is an excellent experience to support the power of connection among people. Yoga is defined as "union," and all the components of yoga stimulate this general principal of unity within oneself, as well as unity with all. The world comes into focus for the child and she feels a stronger desire to know what is happening in the world.

## MULTIDISCIPLINARY

A gentle yoga class provides stimulation in all areas of development. The postures provide an opportunity to hone gross motor skills, including balancing on one leg, and fine motor skills, through the use of mudra, finger lacing and clapping. Speech and language skills are stimulated throughout the session as the child responds to language concepts that are embedded in directions.

In the weight bearing poses of Arch, Cat and Dog, the child develops upper and lower extremity strength. Body awareness is improved through self-guided movement and directionality and crossing arms in front at the midline, and grading or smoothness of movement is rehearsed. Opportunities for weight bearing on the hands strengthens the shoulders, arms and hands for improved fine motor skill. Mudra encourages complex and creative wrist, hand and finger coordination.

The opportunity to relax, self-focus and become in touch with your body and feelings can result in emotional release. Yoga is often a catalyst for inner growth and awareness, and many children benefit from slowing into the yoga mode to better nurture their "soft" side. Overall, yoga impacts all areas of pediatric therapy as it focuses on the total being of each individual.

## SENSORY INTEGRATION

Sensory integration skills are promoted by the practice of therapeutic yoga. Yoga postures provide proprioceptive (impact into the joints and the muscles around the joints), as well as vestibular input (movement through space.) An example of vestibular input is the rocking portion of a spinal roll; and as the child's feet meet the mat in the final upright posture, proprioceptive information is achieved. Both of these stimulations can alert and calm the nervous system of a child with a sensory integration diagnosis. Inversions such as Ragdoll, Gorilla, Windmill and Boulder provide upside-down vestibular stimulation, and Triangle and Sway promote a lateral stretch. A spinal roll incorporates the alerting quality of movement through space, and at the same time stimulates the length of the spine with proprioceptive pressure. The weightbearing involved in Table, Downward dog and Arch send information through the joints and the muscles and tendons around the joints, and provide further proprioceptive information to the child's system.

Yoga therapy incorporates a multitude of inputs to each and every part of the body. The entire physical energetic systems are stimulated and breath is carried to each stretched body part. The thoroughness of the yoga therapy sequence guarantees total body stimulation. Eye bags weighted with flax seeds and lavender blossoms are heated in a microwave oven and used during the final relaxation period of *savasana*. (See correct use of eye bags described on p.122 and the illustration on page 123.) This provides a tactile and weight component to prepare for a state of relaxation. Tucking a blanket around the child further contributes to the goal of relaxation by providing the child greater definition of his body in space and stimulating the nervous system.

## NATURAL SETTING

Therapy support for the special needs child is most widely accepted in a natural setting—in the home, at school, or with a few friends, for instance. These kinds of natural settings allow the child to meet his therapy goals while participating in popular activities in a setting that is typical for him. A home yoga program, a small yoga therapy class in the community that supports family involvement, or a group class incorporated into the school program, are three perfect examples of this. The child is able to share a special activity with family and friends while concurrently experiencing the therapeutic benefits. To develop self-confidence and enjoyment in an activity is not always frequent in the special needs population, and yoga is a beautiful opportunity to participate in a popular practice that is appropriate for everyone.

## MULTIDIMENSIONAL APPROACH

From ancient times, the Hindu community has used yoga to maintain health and well-being. Yoga is a life practice, and in complete use it incorporates spiritual awareness and focus. The yoga program integrates the structural with the energetic to balance and uplift the total being. The intention of yoga is to stimulate and balance on all levels, including physical, mental, emotional and spiritual. It is not uncommon for yoga, in stimulating emotional and mental awareness, to simultaneously awaken the generosity of the spirit.

The added benefit of clearing, integrating and often healing is a more subtle effect of yoga that can be beneficial to a person who has undergone a difficult birth, medical or environmental trauma and/or mental or emotional abuse. How we behave is a manifestation of our inner state of being, and anything that allows us to shift inwardly can result in improved outward choices. Yoga has been found to improve matters of the heart by bringing our awareness to unconditionally loving ourselves. When a child accepts who he is and loves himself, it creates the potential to share that acceptance with every other person around him. In a population where acceptance may not always be prevalent, there is great peace to be found in establishing self-acceptance.

## HEALTHY BODY

The yoga benefits of improved respiration include, as already discussed, oxygenation of the body and brain. There are many other advantages in practicing yoga for supporting a healthier body. When the knees-to-chest posture is practiced, the pressure to the abdomen and the internal organs squeezes out residual blood and allows new blood to circulate into the organs. A sequence of knee-to-chest, first on the right and then on the left, encourages a circular motion of light pressure that aids with natural digestion. This exercise can be helpful to stimulate digestion that has been altered by the intake of medication.

In addition to filtered nasal inhalations and improved respiratory cycles, another benefit of therapeutic yoga is the cleansing of the lungs. This benefit supports healthier respiratory excursions for overall improvement of total respiration.

Postures that include weight bearing build muscle strength, while lengthening poses facilitate flexibility of movement. Bilateral (exercising both sides of the body) use is automatic throughout the protocol, and range of motion is accomplished. A low-tone body builds strength and a high-tone body stretches and relaxes. Yoga therapy can complement all other therapies and activities.

## RESTORATIVE

Many have expounded on the benefits of yoga as a restorative practice. Sam Dworkis (1997) teaches about the restorative powers of yoga and how it helped him regain body function following an automobile accident. Yoga has become a practice that is recommended to rebuild muscle and stimulate weight bearing activity for bone strength, as well as improve bilateral coordination. These areas are targeted in rehabilitation programs which bring the added benefit of reducing anxiety and improving mental attitude.

Because yoga oxygenates the body it is an excellent choice for a gentle cardiac or respiratory rehabilitation program. Elevating the arms overhead strengthens respiration and encourages deeper breathing. When you stretch constricted portions of the body while breathing deeply, you isolate areas you wish to oxygenate.

## SLEEP PATTERNS

Several parents have reported that yoga has improved the sleeping habits of their children. They often explain that their child develops the ability to go to sleep independently and also to sleep for a longer period of time. The parents further report that restlessness is reduced, and as interruptions in sleep decrease, the child becomes more positive about bedtime. The improvement in quantity and quality of sleep supports improved function in all areas of the child's life. Most parents have told me that they function better themselves, as they, too, are more rested and energetic.

## SKILL SET

Probably one of the greatest motivational aspects in yoga is that it builds a skill for each child. Yoga is popular in our society and around the world, and to develop a skill in this practice supports self-esteem. Yoga is not an activity that all children are skilled at, and may provide an opportunity for a child with special needs to shine. With the eventual development of ease in executing yoga poses, added to the development of leadership skills, a child with special needs can learn to share her yoga skills with others.

To become accomplished in a skill and then be able to share it with others is a goal of many people. It is an opportunity to serve and to give back.

## ENERGETIC ALIGNMENT

Yoga balances the energy body by stimulating the seven chakra centers that are housed along the spine, neck and head portions of the body (see Chapter Five). Each yoga pose stimulates one or more of the chakra centers and evokes a greater awareness of the qualities held in that chakra. The intent of a well designed yoga sequence is to purposefully move energy through the body to align the seven chakras while at the same time integrating the energetic body with the physical body.

The seven chakras are discussed more thoroughly in Chapter Five, together with an illustration of their location in the energy body.

# 3

## GETTING READY

To prepare for the first yoga class, it is important to have an in-depth understanding of the child's body and any special needs that may be present. For medically diagnosed children it is important to consult with the child's physician for any special considerations they might recommend. Awareness of anatomy and patterns of physiology are pertinent and knowledge of skeletal, muscular and tendon status is important. With this prerequisite completed you are ready to plan the space where you will practice yoga.

## CREATING A SPACE

The yoga setting is a special place for all who enter. There is a need to feel the difference in this space from that of the hurried world we experience throughout most of our day. The context needs to mirror the goal you have for the child and maintain the simplicity, calm and balanced state of yoga. Designing this space is important if you wish to support your child in creating new skills. A yoga space can be as simple as a yoga mat placed in a quiet corner of the child's bedroom. A more extensive design could be an extra room that is not being used: make it a special place for the whole family to go if they wish to have quiet time for reflection or to do yoga poses. Keep this space special and use it only for yoga-related activities.

In this chapter I seek to support a parent who wishes to create a yoga space in their home. There are many considerations that you can add to make this space more effective.

## Visual simplicity with appeal

The yoga setting is a place where we practice going inside of ourselves, and removing ourselves from outward distractions. For a child who has difficulty calming and eliminating the clutter from the mind, it is crucial that the yoga space be simple, tranquil and clutter-free. The colors are best subdued and soft. Shades of blue, green, yellow or purple can be calming. A few visually soothing additions can be a painting in pastel colors that depicts water or nature. I always keep a plant in my yoga space to provide a piece of nature. Plants also oxygenate the room. Plain mat colors facilitate relaxation. Any item that overstimulates is not appropriate for the yoga space. This space is a backdrop for the inner work a child is moving towards.

## Aromatherapy

Aromatherapy augments yoga by stimulating the olfactory system. I use aromatherapy before, during and at the end of each yoga session. Prior to and throughout the yoga therapy I burn a vanilla-scented candle which promotes relaxation and a calming effect. During the final relaxation and guided imagery, I heat and place lavender-filled eye bags on each child's face (see correct use of eye bags described on p.122). Heating the eye bag increases the scent of lavender. This scent is known for its calming and healing properties. The scent of vanilla lavender facilitate relaxation. Be sure to select fragrances that are known to soothe, and use them sparingly so as not to overstimulate the child.

*Sensory comfort*

A blanket tucked around the child provides input that promotes sensory organization and calming. I use soft lap blankets that are the perfect size for a child. Again, the color should harmonize with the setting, in both color and texture. Often our body temperature decreases when we are in a state of meditation and it is wise to provide warmth for the child.

The fragrance of the eye bags mentioned earlier also provides relaxing sensory input. The weight of the bag can help the child relax. Covering the child's eyes helps him to remove outward visual stimulation and may facilitate an inward picture.

For some children, having their space defined by the yoga mat is comforting, as it provides a visual and tactile parameter of their space.

*Music*

Using music during yoga is an additional source of relaxation and stimulates both hemispheres of the brain. The end desire in a yoga class is that you become totally balanced, integrating the physical, structural body with the energetic body, and balancing the two sides of the physical body. Music can facilitate this goal. There are sections in most music stores that focus on music designed for relaxation.

## WHEN, HOW OFTEN AND FOR HOW LONG?

It is best to practice yoga on an empty stomach. After school, before mealtime, may be a favorable time to begin practicing the yoga program. On the weekend you may find that you enjoy starting your morning with yoga. You and your child will discover the time of day that is best for you.

When you first start practicing the yoga program it may be easiest to complete a portion of the sequence. Select either breathing, mantra and mudra, or the flow of poses. It is also effective to lie down and breathe deeply prior to conducting a guided imagery. Transitioning from one pose to the next becomes fluid, with practice. Once you become familiar with the complete program, the length of a class will not exceed thirty minutes.

I find that three yoga sessions per week is effective to support balance and a sense of peace. The ultimate goal of using the yoga program is to follow the order and complete the entire sequence. Although the program works best from start to finish, it is not harmful to practice isolated poses that are recommended specifically for your child's needs. You may wish to complete one breathing game each day, or teach another game that is recommended in the section for your child's diagnosis.

Regardless of how much time you have to practice the yoga program, it is important that you allow time for *savasana*, or total relaxation, at the end of the session. This is the inward time when the body has an opportunity to integrate all that has been practiced. You can choose to use guided imagery, or simply relax quietly for three to five minutes.

## ASSESSMENT BY OBSERVATION

Observing the child during movement will allow you to note strength, flexibility, range of movement, motor planning, coordination, effectiveness of attention and follow through. Take note of the child's breathing as she carries out the postures and look out for any discomfort in the child throughout the sequence. Let the yoga therapy program be your guide and enjoy the process of beginning this beautiful journey as a team.

## INTRODUCING THE SETTING

Introduce the child to his mat while explaining that yoga mats are also called "sticky mats." This term is used because wherever you place your feet on a yoga mat, the texture and property of the mat provide a quality of grip that allows your feet to stick in place. Explain about taking off socks and shoes because it is important to have bare feet for optimal performance in yoga. Remind the child that loose, comfortable clothing that moves while you are stretching is the best attire for yoga.

# 4

## THE YOGA PROGRAM

### PARADIGM FOR SUCCESS

At this point, I always explain that yoga is a personal activity that looks different with each individual. I also share that the success of yoga is not how we look on the outside, but rather, how we feel on the inside.

You might like to note any observations next to the relevant postures in the following list, or perhaps to record comments directly on a copy of each pose. This may help you to assess your child's present ability to hold a pose, in relation to the target for that posture.

The great advantage of yoga is that it is available and possible for anyone and everyone. Each and every person can participate at their level of capability with no prerequisites other than the ability to breathe in and out. I remember when my yoga teacher, Priscilla Potter, told me that it "would be better to lie on the yoga mat and breathe consciously than to move through any pose while holding your breath." This made a strong impact on me and I have never forgotten that breathing consciously is a big step forward in improving the overall quality of one's life. I also understood that yoga poses without conscious breathing were simply stretches, not yoga. I also learned that improved deep breathing with guided imagery while lying on a yoga mat can be a complete yoga program for a child who can participate only at this level.

## YOGA PROGRAM SEQUENCE

Namasté
Breath work
Tibetan bells
Mudra and mantra
*Savasana* (resting supine)

Postures
Full body stretch
Leg extensions
Supine spinal twist
Arch
Spinal roll to sitting
Forward bend
Table
Volcano
Butterfly breathing with yoga hug
Butterfly
Flower
Sitting spinal twist
Sitting sway pose
Cat
Downward dog
Upward-facing dog
Child's pose
Squat
Standing mountain
Helicopter
Half moon
Half wheel
Umbrella
Triangle
Tree pose
Helicopter
*Savasana* with guided imagery
Closing mudra and mantra
*Namasté*

## NAMASTÉ

### The posture

Sitting in crossed legs position put your hands together, fingers pointing upward, and place them in front of your heart. Your energetic heart spot is in the middle of your chest. Gently bow towards the teacher and say "*namasté (nah-ma-stay)*."

### The benefits

*Namasté* is a greeting of respect and means "I honor the light in you." Another way of saying this is "The light in me sees the light in you." This salutation has been described in a poem:

> I honor the place in you of love and light...
> I honor the place in you where the whole
> universe resides...
> I honor the place in you where—when you are in
> that place in you
> and I am in that place in me—there is only one of us.
>
> Author unknown

*Namasté* sets a mood of respect at the beginning of the yoga session. This greeting acknowledges that we each have a light source within us and supports a universal connection. The child is guided to the heart spot and an opportunity to work in loving.

Hands are placed in midline and a social connection is made, with turn-taking. Eye contact is important, and is facilitated with a motor movement.

### Special considerations

When a child is nonverbal, the opportunity to demonstrate *namasté* through hand posture supports the student's communication at his highest level. A child with one-sided weakness can use his strong hand to bring the weak hand to midline.

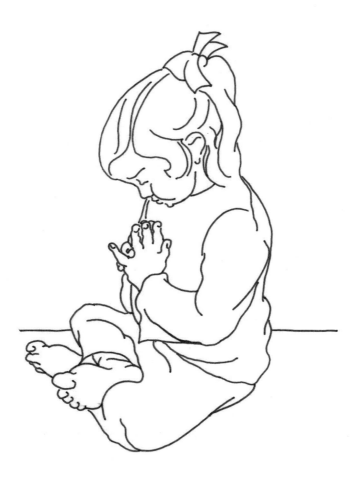

*Namasté*

## BREATH WORK (1): BLOWING BUBBLES

*The posture*

Take a deep and slow breath through your nose. Slowly and gently blow the air through your mouth and return the bubbles that I have blown to you. A long, slow breath will move the bubbles farther than a burst of exhalation.

Now I want you to blow a big bubble. Breathe in deeply through your nose and then gently and slowly blow into the bubble wand and make a large bubble. (Feel the slow exhalation as I blow on your hand. This is how your breath will feel when you breathe in deeply and blow the breath out slowly.)

*The benefits*

As you blow bubbles to the child, remember to encourage them to breathe in through their nose and breathe out through their mouth. Many children have not been taught how to breathe and have not experienced a deep inhalation with sustained exhalation. The benefit of blowing bubbles for respiratory practice is twofold—the child receives visual feedback while also engaging in a playful activity. Once the child has accomplished blowing a large bubble, they experience the sensation of graded exhalation. This control of breath may take months to achieve, but once they have established the sensation of grading, they generally do not regress.

Mastering deeper inhalation with graded exhalation necessitates a near closed mouth posture. The child becomes more aware of the posture of the oral mechanism during breathing, as well as of the quality of the breath. This new awareness and skill prepares the child for sustained, graded respiration for more effective oxygenation of the body—as well as for physical endurance and speech production. A stronger respiratory cycle also supports a healthier body.

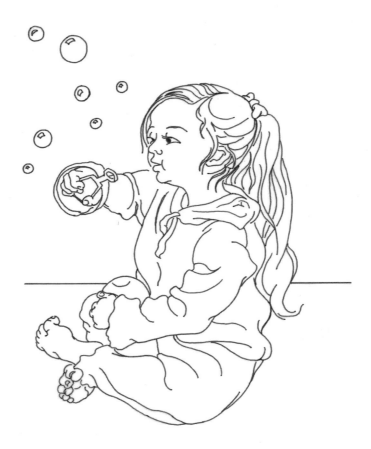

*Breathing (1)*

If you are teaching in a small group, guide the children to take turns with one another, blowing large bubbles or blowing them back to a partner.

One of the benefits of improved respiration is the opportunity to move into deeper states of relaxation and to achieve this transition more quickly.

## Special considerations

For a child who is demonstrating great difficulty with breathing more deeply or who cannot sustain the exhalation, counting is often helpful. Count as the child inhales a breath, and then ask them to exhale for the same length of count. This can provide a greater understanding of how the inhalation and exhalation correlate. If a child is unable to blow bubbles, you can blow a bubble and catch it on the wand. Then place your wand in front of the child's mouth and ask him to blow softly. The child will benefit from observing how far his bubble will float without popping. A softer, more sustained exhalation will send the bubble further and it will retain its shape longer.

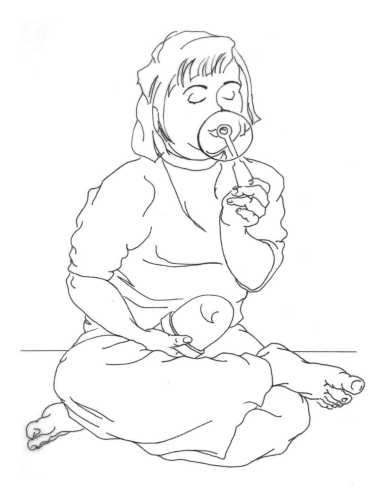

*Breathing (2)*

## BREATH WORK (2): ALTERNATE NOSTRIL BREATHING

*The posture*

Bend your index finger and middle finger into the palm of your hand, leaving only the ring finger, baby finger and thumb extended. Now place your thumb against your nose and close off your right nostril. Breathe in through your left nostril. Then place your ring finger on your left nostril. Lift your thumb off your right nostril, and slowly exhale out of your right nostril. With your ring finger still closing your left nostril, breathe in through your right nostril. Now press your thumb on your right nostril, lift your ring finger off the left nostril, and exhale out of your left nostril. Breathe in through your left nostril and close it off with your ring finger. Lift your thumb off your right nostril and exhale slowly through the right nostril. Repeat three more times.

*The benefits*

This breathing exercise is designed to take the child into deeper breathing than they were experiencing with the bubble-blowing activity. Alternate nostril breathing allows the child to direct the breath more specifically and to control a deeper inhalation, and ultimately a longer exhalation.

This breathing technique quickly oxygenates the entire body and creates a state of increased alertness while concurrently bringing more peace.

*Special considerations*

Children learn to breathe more smoothly when practicing in front of the teacher. Be sure the child is never holding his breath and physically guide him through the finger releases, if needed.

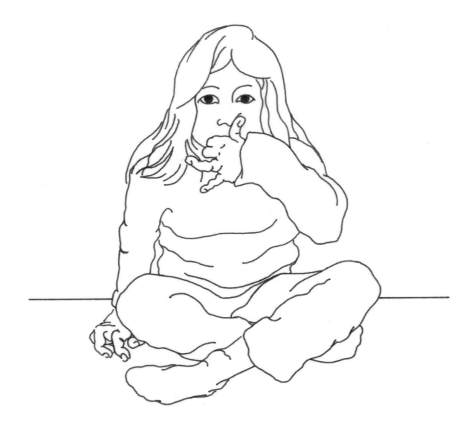

*Alternate nostril breathing*

## TIBETAN BELLS

*The posture*

Pick up the bells with two hands and pinch the cord with your fingers. Hold your arms up in front of you and gently move the bells together until they ring. Wait until you can no longer hear the bell tone and gently place them on the floor.

*The benefits*

The gentle ringing of the bells encourages a calm mood and offers another opportunity for active participation. Pincer grasp is encouraged. This activity requires bilateral participation, graded movement to midline, and arms extended up against gravity. Listening to the tone provides auditory awareness. Gentle ringing of the bells requires grading of movement and awareness of the quality that is sought. The weight of the bells augments strength building when the arms are extended. The weight is also grounding for those children with sensory integration needs.

*Special considerations*

Students unable to execute pincer grasp may use a two-fisted grip. The student who does not have fine grading may hear a loud or dull ring. The auditory result of ringing the bells provides the child with feedback for moving towards a softer tone, and thus finer grading.

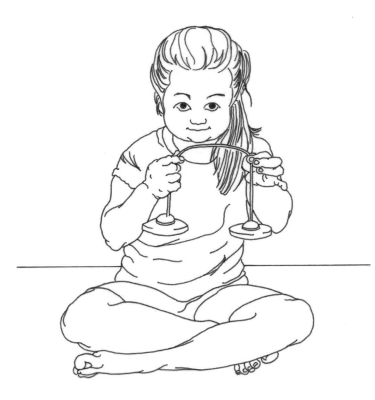

*Tibetan bells*

## MUDRA AND MANTRA

*The posture*

Form the OM mudra with both hands by making a circle with the thumb and index finger. Place the back of your hands on your knees with your palms facing upward. Chant "OM" for 20 seconds. Our voices blend as one.

*The benefits*

*Mudra* is the Sanskrit word for the mystical hand gestures that represent the symbolic language of yoga. The various placements of hands and fingers are used to redirect energy from the hands into the spinal column and to stimulate the chakra centers (see Chapter Five) for greater outward radiance. These postures are also used to communicate moods without using words, a bit like sign language.

*Mantra* is the term for the chants used in yoga to center oneself. The mantras are simple and easy to chant, allowing any child the opportunity for success. For those who are not vocal or verbal, mudra and mantra provide a mode of communication. They also encourage sequenced motor planning.

*Special considerations*

If a child is new to the setting, she is not requested to take a turn leading the group. For a child who is not vocal or verbal, the accompanying mudra is a mode by which to participate. For children with poor sequencing skills and/or poor fine motor skills, the mantra and mudra combinations are varied in difficulty, and the simplest level can be initiated.

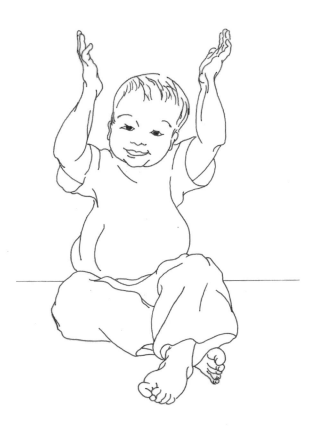

*Mudra and mantra*

## SAVASANA (RESTING SUPINE)

*The posture*

Lie on your back with your legs stretched out, arms resting away from your sides and the palms of your hands facing up. Be sure your feet are active, with the toes pointed to the ceiling. Breathe in through your nose and gently let the breath out through your mouth.

*The benefits*

Lying on his back, the child has the opportunity to relax. At this time he is practicing the optimal breath for yoga without the added skill of moving into a posture. This preparatory pose helps him get in touch with his body and have a moment of silence prior to moving into further yoga poses.

*Special considerations*

If the child complains of low back pain, have him bend both knees and gently move them together for support.

For the child with extensor pattern of the feet, remind her that wherever she is able to bend her ankles for upward toes, that is perfect.

If a child exhibits a pronounced extension of the head, encourage her to bring her chin to her chest and then relax into this new posture. If this does not facilitate greater neck flexion, you can place a firm, thin massage pillow under her head for improved alignment.

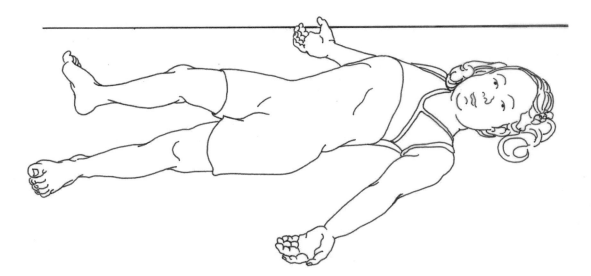

*Savasana*

## FULL BODY STRETCH

*The posture*

Inhale through your nose as you raise both arms over your head, and rest them above your head on the mat. Breathe deeply through your nose and let the breath out slowly through your mouth. Stretch your body long, and then relax. Inhale through your nose again, and as you slowly let your breath out, lower your arms back down by your sides.

*The benefits*

This pose allows a deep breath to be taken into the body while it is fully lengthened and aligned. Oxygenation occurs throughout the body as the student practices his inhalation with extension.

The language concepts of "above" and "by" are practiced, while facilitating the opportunity for lung expansion. As in all yoga poses, bilateral movement is requested. The shoulder joints are gently stretched, and the back lengthens.

*Special considerations*

For children with tight shoulder joints or contraction, any overhead extension of the arms is acceptable. It may be necessary to extend one arm at a time. Children with lower back problems can bend their knees, lift their buttocks, and gently press their back into the mat, keeping their knees bent through the arm stretch. This will relieve stress to the back.

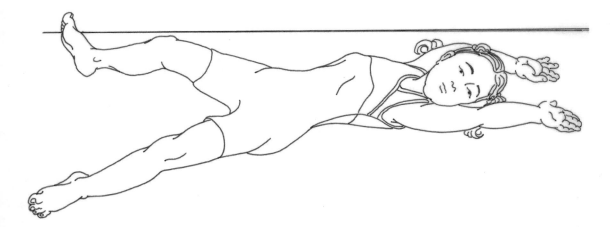

*Full body stretch*

## LEG EXTENSIONS

### The posture

Bend your knees and place both feet on the mat. Breathe in through your nose, and as you let the breath out, bend your right knee into your chest and hold your knee with both hands. As you breathe in, stretch your right leg to the ceiling, hold your leg up with both hands placed on the back of your thigh, and point your toes. Now push your heel to the ceiling, and then point your toes. Again, push your heel and point your toe. Now wiggle your toes, pretending you are waving to the ceiling. Make a small circle with your big toe and move your ankle in circles. Take a deep, slow breath, and as you let your breath out, bend your knee to your chest. Breathe in through your nose, and as you breathe out, lift your head to your knee. Relax your back, neck and head on the mat, and place your right foot on the mat. Repeat on the left.

### The benefits

The overall benefit of this series of stretches is to provide full range of motion from the hip to the toes. Circulation increases and any tightness to the hip, knee, ankle or toe joints may relax. The muscles are also stretched, including the gluteus, back quadriceps, hamstrings and Achilles tendon.

Language concepts of *up*, *point*, *push*, *around* and *circle* are practiced.

As in all yoga postures, the breath is guided through the natural patterns of extension and flexion. The head to knee position of the stretch provides flexion of the trunk and facilitates lengthening of the cervical and upper thoracic spine.

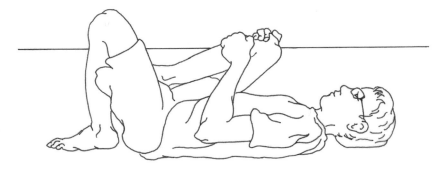

*Knee to chest*

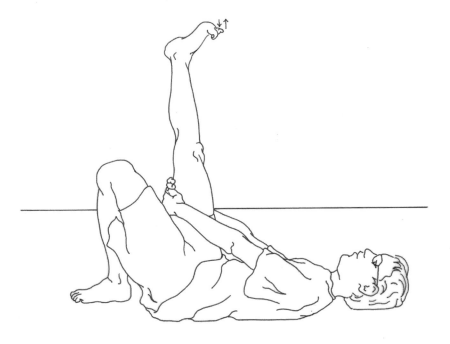

*Extended leg wiggle toes*

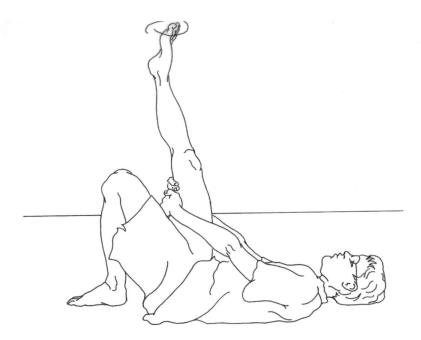

*Extended leg, circle ankle*

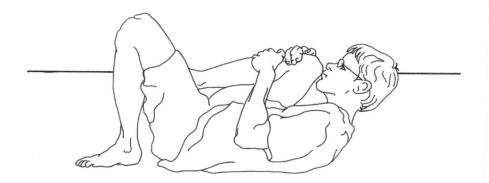

*Head to knee*

*Special considerations*

A child with tight hamstrings may not demonstrate a full extension of the leg. This may cause a natural desire to lift the head to compensate. Encourage the student to relax his back, neck and head on the mat.

Tight Achilles tendons may result in the child not being able to push his heel to the ceiling. Encourage the child to move his body only to a limit that is comfortable for him.

For children lacking flexible ankle mobility, the circle they make with the big toe may result in a full leg circle. Demonstrate moving the ankle so that the foot internally rotates, and then externally rotates. Again, this circle may be difficult for children who have a pattern of internal or external rotation of the foot.

With children under the age of nine, I change the directions for bringing their head to their knee. I ask them to kiss their knee, and they achieve excellent flexion.

## SUPINE SPINAL TWIST

*The posture*

> With your knees bent and your feet on the floor, place your knees together and your ankles together, and put your arms out to your sides like angel wings. Take a breath through your nose and drop your knees to the right. Be sure to keep your shoulders flat on the mat, and turn your head as far as you can to the left. Breathe in through your nose and breathe out. Inhale and lift your knees to the middle, at the same time as you turn your head to look straight up at the ceiling. Let your breath out slowly as you drop your bent knees to the left, and turn your head as far as you can to the right. Breathe in through your nose and breathe out. Inhale as you move your knees to the middle, and turn your head so that you are once again looking at the ceiling.

*The benefits*

> Supine spinal twist allows separation of the pelvic girdle and the shoulder girdle. Rotation provides a stretch to those muscles attached to the sacrum (the base of the spine, above the tail bone).
>
> Motor planning with rotation of the body is practiced, at the same time as coordination of the breath. Left and right directionality is practiced with body awareness.

*Special considerations*

> For children who are lifting their back off the mat, it may be helpful to tell them to keep their back flat.
>
> It is important to remind the children that it is not important how far their legs rotate, but to keep breathing wherever the rotation is comfortable.
>
> Some children may be more comfortable with their palms facing down on the mat.

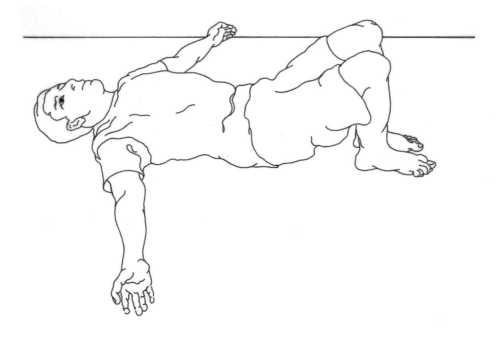

*Supine spinal twist (1)*

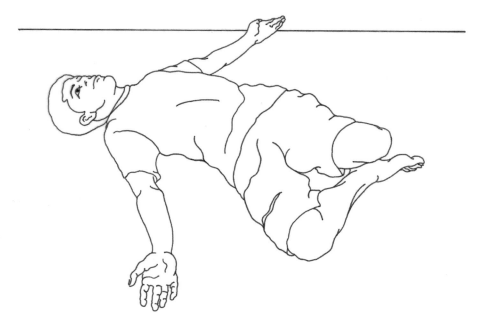

*Supine spinal twist (2)*

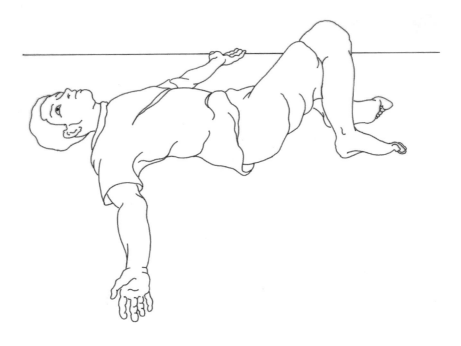

*Supine spinal twist (3)*

## ARCH

*The posture*

Keep your knees bent and move your feet apart. Place your arms by your sides with your palms down. Breathe in and keep your head relaxed and your feet on the mat. Lift your bottom and back off the mat while letting your breath out. Breathe. Hold. Slowly roll your back down onto the mat, beginning at the shoulders, one vertebra at a time.

*The benefits*

Arch provides flexion of the neck while providing extension of the lower back. This pose strengthens the buttocks and the legs and encourages respiration in a posture where the child might normally hold his breath.

*Special considerations*

A child with low tone may find it difficult to hold the pose for more than a few seconds. Encourage the child to go back into the pose and count beyond the point where she was previously able to hold the position: if the pose was held for five seconds on a previous trial, encourage her now to hold it for the count of six. If a child is having difficulty lifting more than a few inches off the mat, encourage her by telling her a boat is coming under her bridge and it needs to get through. This game generally encourages a higher lift.

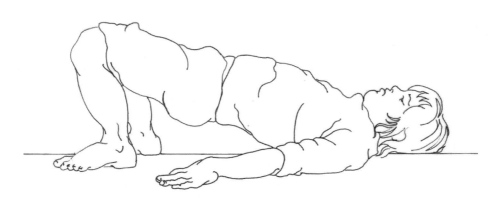

*Arch*

## SPINAL ROLL TO SITTING

*The posture*

Breathe in as you roll backwards and bring both knees to your chest. Bring your head up and forward while swinging your legs up to a sitting position. Roll back with speed, and again roll forward into sitting. Depending on the child's momentum their knees may come up on either side of their head as they roll backwards. Repeat this three more times.

*The benefits*

Spinal roll provides total body flexion. When rolling backwards and forwards, the spine is massaged and it is allowed to gently align.

The movement in spinal roll stimulates the vestibular system, alerts the nervous system, and provides proprioceptive input to the spine. With enough momentum, the soles of the feet also stimulate proprioception as they hit the mat on sitting up.

*Special considerations*

Many children have low tone trunks and weak abdominals, and the speed of the movement will help them roll back up into sitting until their abdominal muscles and trunk are stronger. For those who cannot achieve the momentum and strength to roll upwards, the teacher provides support behind the upper back and gently lifts and directs the movement forward.

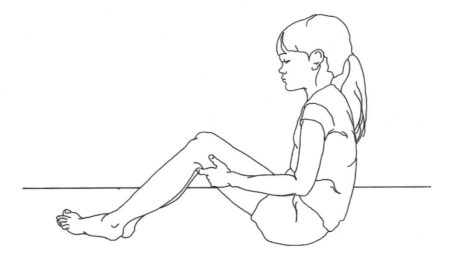

*Spinal roll (1)*

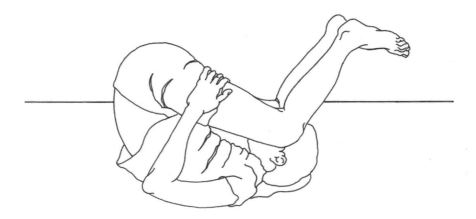

*Spinal roll (2)*

## FORWARD BEND

### The posture

Straighten your legs out in front of you and place them together. Be sure your toes are pointed upward for active yoga feet. Sit tall and bend forward over your legs. Hold, and breathe in through your nose and slowly out through your mouth. Feel your back relax as you hold this pose and continue to breathe slowly.

### The benefits

Forward bend allows extension of the legs while stretching the buttocks, hamstrings and Achilles tendon. The upper body relaxes into gravity and a position of flexion. The relaxed head posture provides elongation of the cervical spine, and there is a gentle elongation of the entire spine.

### Special considerations

Often a child with tight hamstrings and/or Achilles tendons will bend her knees and externally rotate her legs. This defeats the stretch to the lower body, and her legs need to be realigned. It is important to be sitting upright on the sit bones during this pose. With a tighter body the child may not be able to bend forward very far. Remind her that the bend should be comfortable, and that she is perfect right where she is.

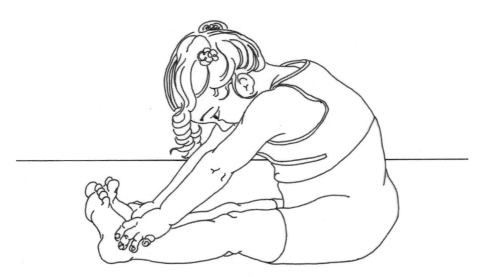

*Forward bend*

## TABLE

*The posture*

Bend your knees and move your feet apart. Put your hands behind you, with your fingers pointing towards your feet. Lift your buttocks and make the front of your body flat like a table. Tilt your head back in alignment with your body. At this time, I encourage the child to hold the position until he has finished telling me what he is "serving" on his table.

*The benefits*

This posture strengthens both the upper and lower extremities as well as the buttocks. It is a balance pose that additionally provides weightbearing. The creative sharing about what is being served on the table encourages creative language, turn taking, information on the child's favorite foods as well as taking their mind off the muscle burn they may be feeling.

*Special considerations*

The pose may not be held long by a child with low body tone or upper extremity weakness. Encourage this child to rest and try it again. This pose is difficult, but not impossible, for a child with unilateral weakness. Motor planning for this position teaches a child how to bear weight on the arms.

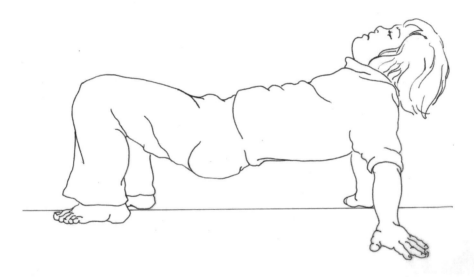

*Table*

## VOLCANO

*The posture*

Sitting with your legs crossed in front of you and a tall back, place your hands in *namasté*. Breathe in as you slowly raise your hands up past your face and as high as you can. Be sure your palms are together throughout this part of the pose. Spread your arms out in a wide arc as you exhale, and slowly bring them down and back into *namasté*. Repeat this exercise and complete with your hands in *namasté*.

*The benefits*

Full arm extension is achieved with this pose as the shoulders are exercised through their full range of movement, and the child learns how to move up through midline and outward into lateral excursion.

Coordination of breathing is practiced with a natural flow. Low tone children will benefit from strengthening of the arms by moving them up against gravity. The spine is lengthened and strengthened.

*Special considerations*

The child with hemiparesis is provided an opportunity for the strong arm and hand to facilitate the weaker side into full extension. If a child does not reach high, encourage her to move her fingertips to the ceiling.

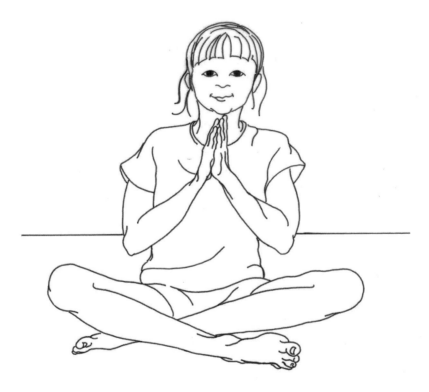

*Namasté*

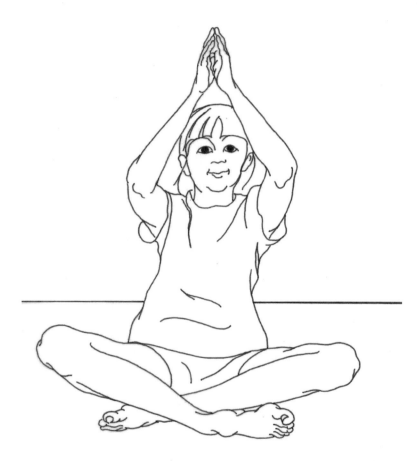

*Volcano (1)*

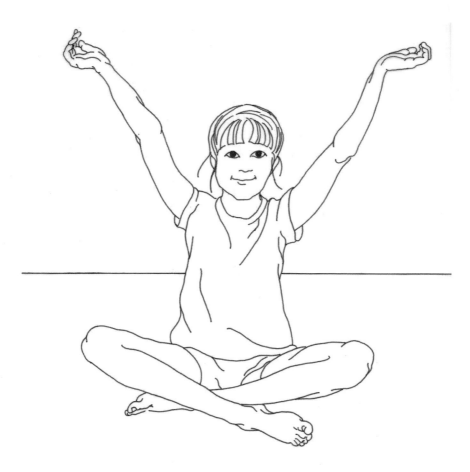

*Volcano (2)*

## BUTTERFLY BREATHING WITH YOGA HUG

*The posture*

With your hands in *namasté*, stretch your arms out as far as you can in front of you. Now you are taking your love out into the world. Breathe in as you move your hands apart and spread your arms out to the side as far as they can go. Breathe out as you move your arms back together in front of you and place your hands together. Repeat this one more time. Next, breathe in and move your arms out to the side, and then, as you bring the arms back to the front, cross the right arm over the left into a yoga hug. Hold, and breathe in and out as you hug yourself. Breathe in again as you move your arms out to your sides, and then bring them forward again, breathing out as you cross your left arm over your right arm into yoga hug. Hold, and breathe in and out. Breathe in as you move your arms out to the side, and breathe out as you move your arms forward and your hands back together in the middle. Bring your hands into your heart spot in *namasté* and take a full breath.

*The benefits*

Breathing deeply is exaggerated by the wide movement of arms out to the side. Maintaining arms parallel to the floor builds strength while they are up against gravity. This posture provides flexion and extension of the chest and back, and the shoulder blades glide over the back as the arms open wide.

The yoga hug accentuates chest flexion and motor planning for crossing the midline. The general theme of this pose is one of opening the heart, and it teaches the child that loving of self is accepted and important in a yoga practice. Graded movements are emphasized as you ask the child to move her arms gently and slowly, like the elegant wings of a butterfly.

*Special considerations*

Children with weak upper extremities may at first need to stabilize their upper arms against their trunk. If a child has difficulty crossing midline, encourage her by first placing one arm across to the alternate shoulder. Then place the second arm across midline onto the opposite shoulder. Guiding the child is easier from behind when placing one arm gently over the other.

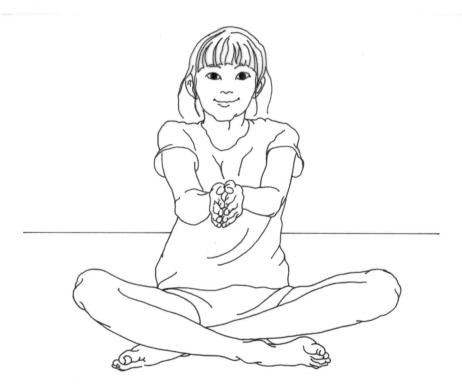

*Namasté out into the world*

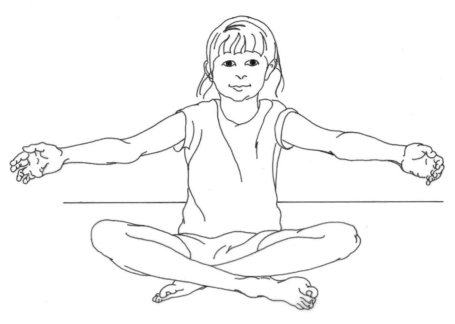

*Butterfly breathing (1)*

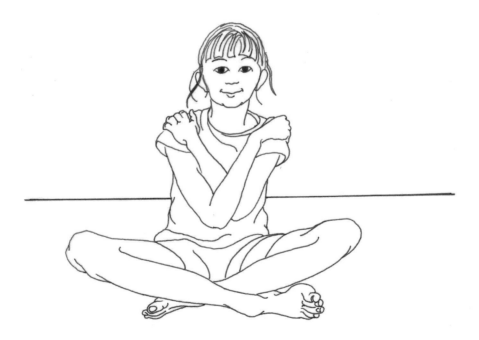

*Yoga hug (1), right over left*

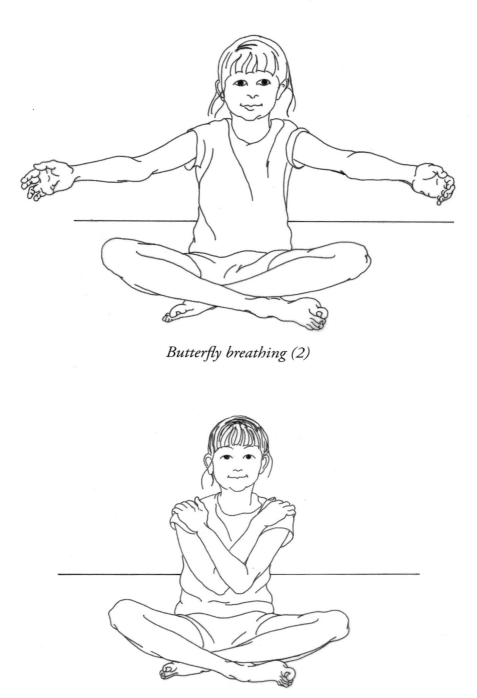

*Butterfly breathing (2)*

*Yoga hug (2), left over right*

## BUTTERFLY

### *The posture*

Sitting with your legs crossed in front of you, open your legs wider and place the soles of your feet together. Move your legs closer or further from your body to find a comfortable placement. Fold your hands over the toes of both feet. If you can lace your fingers together, it can be helpful. Gently move your legs up and down like the wings of a butterfly.

### *The benefits*

The feet are placed at midline. The movement of the legs works the hip joints to create more flexibility. Lacing the fingers requires fine motor control and greater stability for the pose. The inner thighs are stretched. Children with low tone might choose w-sitting (with the lower legs folded outwards to the sides, instead of inward in the cross-legged sitting posture). Sitting with legs crossed requires the low tone child to work their abdominals, whereas w-sitting does not do this.

### *Special considerations*

Some children may have difficulty with the fine motor task of lacing fingers, and a hand-over-hand grip will still encourage midline placement. For children with high tone, the legs may move very little. Those with low tone can be asked to move their knees further upward and off the mat to encourage internal rotation.

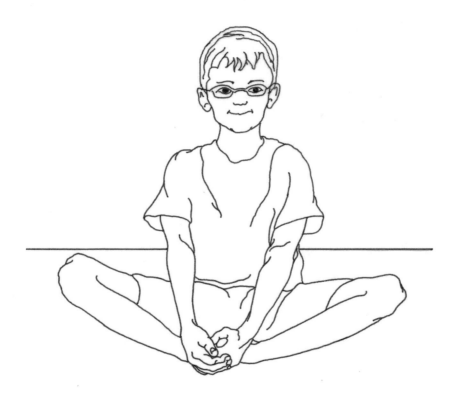

*Butterfly (1)*

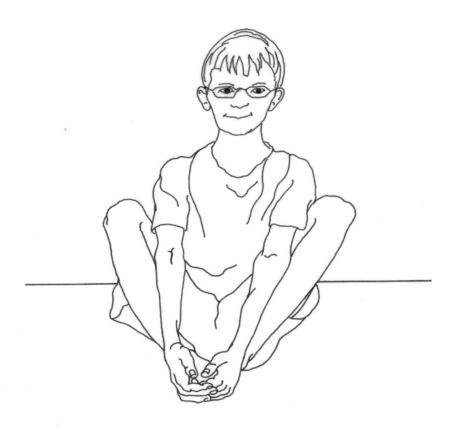

*Butterfly (2)*

## FLOWER

### The posture

Keeping your knees bent, place both feet on the mat, about two feet apart. Put your arms between your legs and scoop under your right leg with your right arm and under your left leg with your left arm. Gently roll back in this position and balance. While you balance here, describe what kind and color of flower you are and what color butterfly has landed on you. Gently roll forward on your feet and bring your arms out from under your legs.

### The benefits

Flower encourages bilateral motor planning. This is a balance pose that encourages the child to balance flexion and extension of the trunk. Breathing deepens to support greater balance. Language is imaginative, with the description of the flower and the butterfly. The communication makes a connection between the poses of Butterfly and Flower for a more natural sequence.

### Special considerations

As in all poses of yoga, the non-verbal child is able to communicate with the posture where words are not yet developed. For a child with low weight or weak abdominals, balance on the sacrum may be difficult. This posture prepares motor planning for eventual movement into balance.

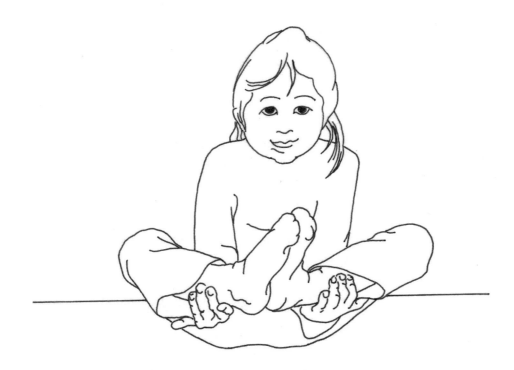

*Flower*

## SITTING SPINAL TWIST

### The posture

Sit with your legs crossed in front of you and place your fingertips out by your sides. Sitting tall, lift your arms up like angel wings and twist your body to the right. Put your left hand on the outside of your right knee and your right hand gently behind you, with fingertips barely resting on the floor. Sit tall and breathe. Lift your arms and twist back to the front, and bring your arms down by your sides. Now breathe your arms back up and twist to the left. Put your right hand on the outside of your left knee and your left hand behind you, with fingertips gently resting on the floor. Sit tall and breathe. Lift your arms and twist back to the front, and breathe your arms back down.

### The benefits

Sitting spinal twist strengthens the arms as they are held up against gravity. The twist provides rotation to the body, and separation of the pelvic and shoulder girdles. The twist also provides a massage to the internal organs. Directionality is practiced, as well as the exercise of crossing midline. Sitting in the cross-legged position encourages trunk stability. (Low tone children may choose w-sitting.)

### Special considerations

Ask the child who has any spinal limitations to twist gently, slowly, and never into a range of pain.

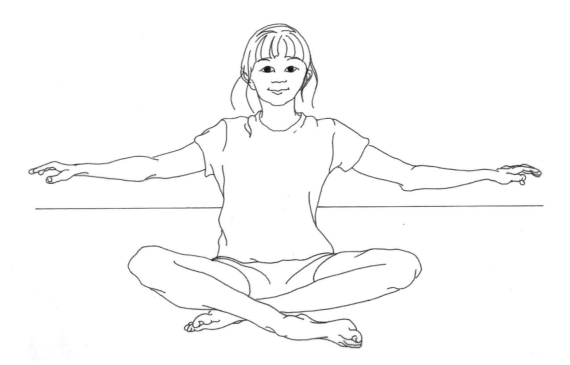

*Sitting spinal twist (1)*

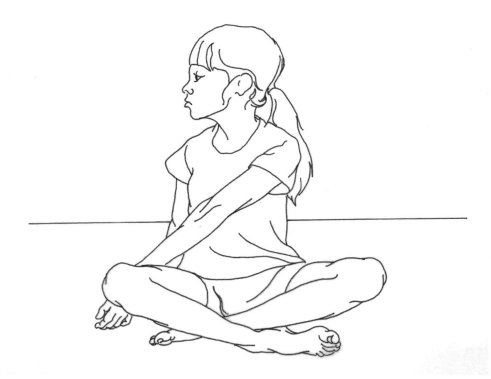

*Sitting spinal twist (2)*

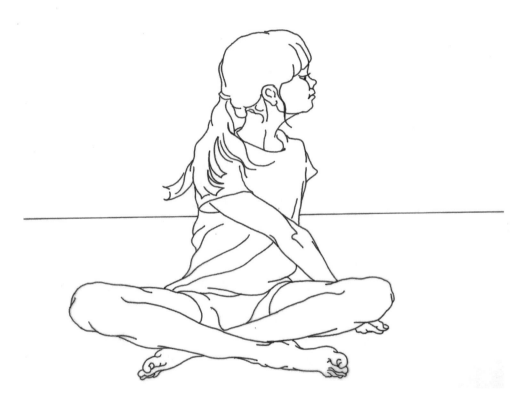

*Sitting spinal twist (3)*

## SITTING SWAY POSE

### The posture

Remain sitting, with legs crossed in front of you. Inhale, moving your arms up over your head, and lace your fingers above you. Push your palms up to the ceiling. Now place your laced fingers behind your head and keep your elbows out to the side. Breathe in, and as you breathe out, sway to the right, making the left side of your body long. Breathe in and out. Breathe in as you move back to a tall sitting posture. Breathe out and sway to the left, making the right side of your body long. Breathe in and out, slowly and deeply. Breathe in and move back to a tall sitting posture. Relax your hands and bring your arms down to your sides.

### The benefits

Sway pose moves the arms against gravity and provides strengthening, as well as a full stretch to the shoulders and arms. Lacing fingers and placing the hands behind the head exercises motor planning skills with fine motor coordination.

Swaying in this pose requires lateral movement that elongates the side of the trunk and stretches the intercostal muscles between the ribs.

Left and right directionality are practiced in this pose, and extension of the upper back is possible.

Pushing palms to the ceiling encourages coordination and flexibility of the wrists.

### Special considerations

Children who are not able to coordinate laced fingers can keep their elbows up with one hand on top of the other. Those who have not yet mastered the ability to rotate the wrists and extend palms upward may unlace their fingers to push their palms upward.

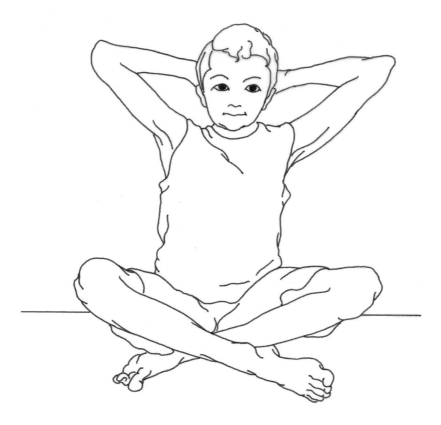

*Sway pose (1)*

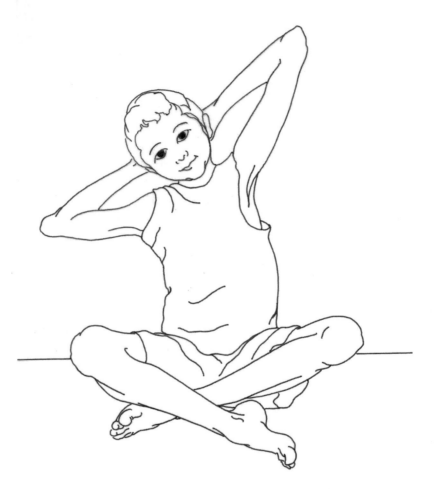

*Sway pose (2)*

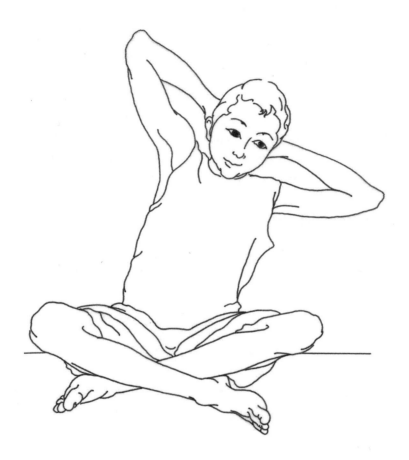

*Sway pose (3)*

## CAT

### The posture

Move onto hands and knees, with your hands under your shoulders and your knees under your hips. Spread your fingers out wide like the paws of a cat. Breathe in as you lift your head up and arch your back. You will look like a swayback horse. Now breathe out as you tuck your head down and arch your back like a Halloween cat. Tighten your stomach as you arch your back. Repeat this sequence.

### The benefits

This posture allows creative expression for the children as we purr and meow and imagine that we are cats. Weightbearing on hands and knees strengthens the arms and encourages even distribution of weight through all the limbs. Hand placement with fingers splayed provides a wider base of support, and practices wrist extension. The arching and rounding of the back exercises and aligns the spine. The rounding of the back also strengthens the abdominals.

### Special considerations

A child with one-sided weakness has the opportunity to stretch the fingers on her weak hand, and to balance some weight onto her weak side, with the support of the stronger side. For a child with weak upper extremities, cat pose provides an opportunity to strengthen the arms while using stronger lower extremities (hip joints all the way down to the toes) for an added base of support.

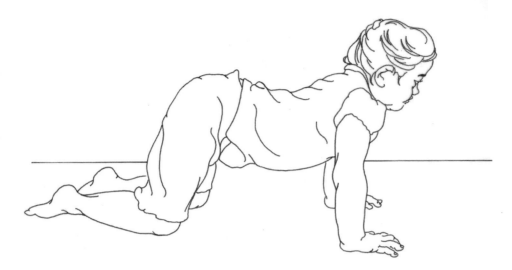

*Cat pose (1)*

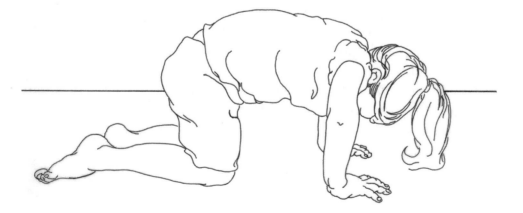

*Cat pose (2)*

## DOWNWARD DOG

### The posture

On hands and knees, keep your hands where they are, curl your toes under and push up on your feet, straightening your legs. Push your buttocks up and straighten your back. Then bring your heels down as close to the mat as is comfortable. Hold, breathe in through your nose and out through your mouth. Remain in Downward dog to make the transition into upward dog.

### The benefits

Downward dog pose strengthens the arms, stretches the Achilles tendons while flexing the ankles, and realigns the spine. Barking and whining like a canine adds the potential for imaginative play. Whimpering, growling and panting allow the child various creative modes of emotional expression. This pose is an inversion and allows the heart reversed gravitational pull, circulating more blood to the upper portion of the body and head.

### Special considerations

A child with upper extremity or unilateral weakness may need to hold the pose briefly, rest and come up into the pose a second time.

Children with tight Achilles tendons may need to widen the stance of their feet for greater ease in bringing their heels to the mat. Be sure the child's head is aligned with his back.

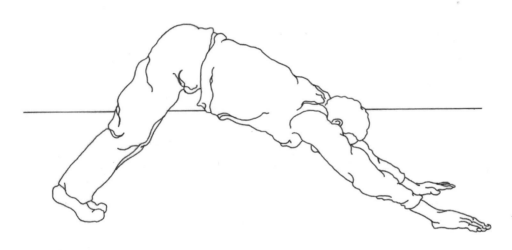

*Downward dog*

## UPWARD-FACING DOG

*The posture*

From Downward dog, move your body forward over your arms and place your legs and stomach on the yoga mat. Uncurl your toes and extend your feet. Push upward on your arms and look up towards the ceiling. Breathe.

*The benefits*

This pose facilitates back extension while also encouraging chest expansion. Arm strength is stimulated as the child's body moves over their arms. The length of the pose encourages elongation of the upper body and extension of the ankles.

*Special considerations*

For a child who is not able to move into this degree of back extension, moving down onto their forearms reduces the range of extension. (This would then become Cobra pose, and instead of barking they would need to hiss like a snake.)

If Cobra pose is used instead of upward-facing dog, there is no weightbearing on the arms, but the benefit of extension is still present and primarily focused between the shoulderblades. For many children who are low in tone, back rounding or hunched sitting can be a compensation that ultimately becomes a structural deviancy. Working with Cobra pose and ultimately moving into upward-facing dog establishes back extension and benefits the low tone child.

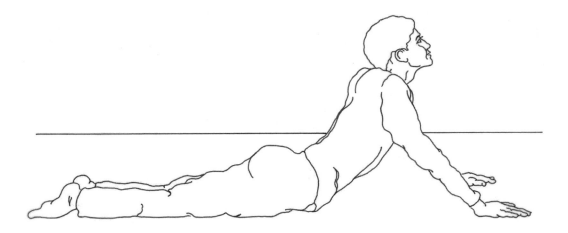

*Upward-facing dog*

## CHILD'S POSE

*The posture*

From hands and knees, sit back on your feet with your toes pointed and relaxed. Bend forward and place your forehead on the mat, wrapping your arms back around your body. Rest your hands and arms on the mat, letting them totally relax into the pose. Breathe and relax.

*The benefits*

Child's pose facilitates foot and ankle extension, with the weight of the body resting on the legs. Complete flexion of the body is established, and a folding of the skeletal frame. Neck elongation is accomplished through proper head placement.

*Special considerations*

For children with poor foot and ankle extension it may be necessary to place a soft therapy roll or rolled up blanket under their ankles to provide support and comfort. If a child has poor head placement she may fall into a pattern of hyperextension of the head. Encourage the child to tuck her chin in and help her place the point of contact higher on the forehead. The folding of the body allows the organs to be compressed, encouraging oxygenation through the vascular cycle of circulation.

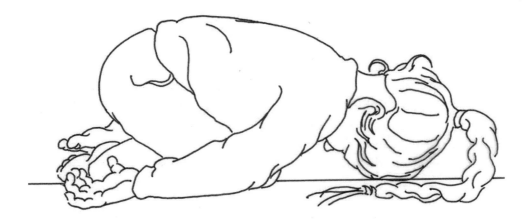

*Child's pose*

## SQUAT

### *The posture*

From the hands and knees position, curl your toes under and push up into a squat. Experiment with the distance between your feet to see where you are most comfortable. Look straight ahead and keep a focus on one spot to help you keep your balance. Breathe deeply. Placing your hands in *namasté* may help you balance this pose. If you are having difficulty balancing, move back onto your knees and widen your stance. If this does not support greater balance, experiment with where you place your hands: rest your elbows on your knees, or possibly move your hands higher in the air. Begin to breathe more deeply as you change your base of support.

### *The benefits*

Squat provides another opportunity to stretch the Achilles tendons, while also maintaining visual focus for balance. Placing the hands in *namasté* brings focus to midline, which facilitates core balance. Deeper breathing and visual focus helps the child who has difficulty with attention and focus.

### *Special considerations*

Some children find it hard to balance in squat. If Achilles tendons are tight, this may be more difficult. A small wedge or a folded yoga blanket can be placed under their heels to provide a greater base of support for balance.

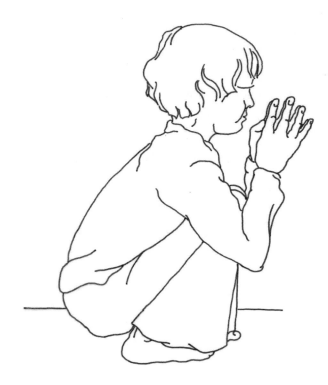

*Squat*

## STANDING MOUNTAIN

*The posture*

Stand up and place your feet under your hips with approximately six inches between them. Keep your knees relaxed and your buttocks tucked under you as you lift the front hip bones upward. Lift your shoulders up, roll them back, and let them fall into a relaxed posture. Keep your head up with your eyes focused forwards. Breathe.

*The benefits*

Standing Mountain pose is anatomically correct standing. When this pose has been aligned properly it is comfortable to stand, as the weight is distributed equally over both legs. Breathing is easier and the entire body is comfortable and relaxed. Teaching this pose helps children be more aware of their standing posture when waiting in line, watching an activity, or simply stretching their legs.

*Special considerations*

Standing Mountain pose is a posture that will generally require input from the yoga therapist. Facilitating a gentle lifting of the belly can totally recreate the comfort of this pose. Seek input from the child and find the spot where she is most comfortable.

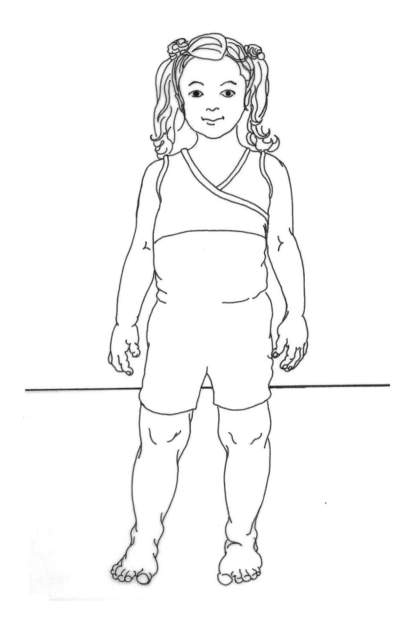

*Standing mountain*

## HELICOPTER

### The posture

First move into Standing Mountain pose. Then, with arms hanging limp at your sides and knees gently bent, begin to twist your body to the right, and then to the left. Let your arms swing around your body and even tap onto your hips as you turn. When you turn to the right, let your left knee rotate inward towards the right side of your body. Do the same with a left twist, letting the right knee gently turn towards the left. This protects the lower vertebrae, which do not rotate on a hinge.

### The benefits

Helicopter realigns the spine, while also providing vestibular stimulation. This spinning posture can be observed in some special needs children outside of the yoga setting, and has been thought to be a relaxing and reorienting experience for them. The Helicopter further allows the practice of maintaining balance while shifting weight from one foot to the other.

### Special considerations

Children with low tone often begin this pose by fixing and remain tight throughout the shoulder girdle and arms. Some children need to be reminded of the importance of bending the knees and following through with knee rotation on the twist. Explain this by providing an example they are familiar with, such as the swinging of a baseball bat.

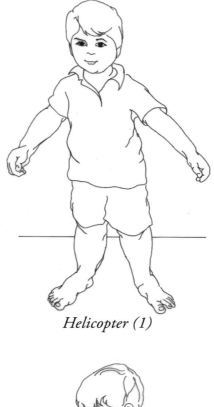

*Helicopter (1)*

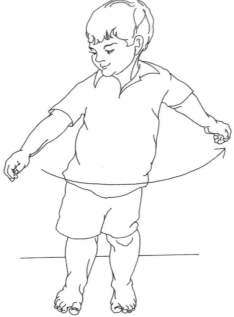

*Helicopter (2)*

## HALF MOON

### The posture

Stand in Mountain pose with your feet slightly apart, stomach tucked in, shoulders back and your arms relaxed. Breathe as you move your arms up over your head with your hands facing one another. Breathe out as you lean to the right with extended arms. Breathe in as you raise your body back to the middle. Breathe out and lean to the left with your arms still extended. Breathe in as you slowly bring your body back to the middle.

### The benefits

Half moon posture provides an opportunity for the full range of arm extension and a lateral stretch through the entire torso. This posture stimulates an upward and lateral expansion of the ribs as they follow the shoulders, stretching the muscles of inhalation. The concept of lateral movement is gained as the child imitates the sideway movement.

### Special considerations

It is important that the child is not locking her elbows, but rather gently curving them for overall fluidity of movement. The placement of the hands, palms inward, creates a deeper stretch than if they are held with the palms forward.

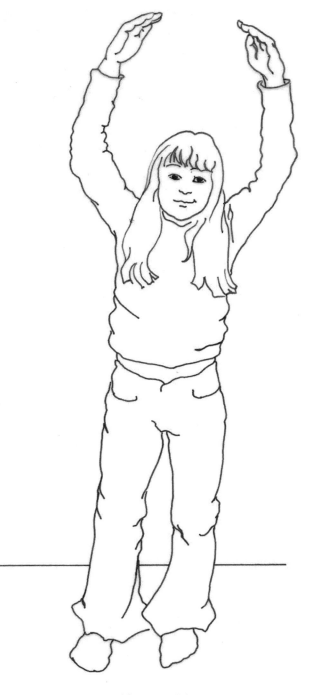

*Half moon (1)*

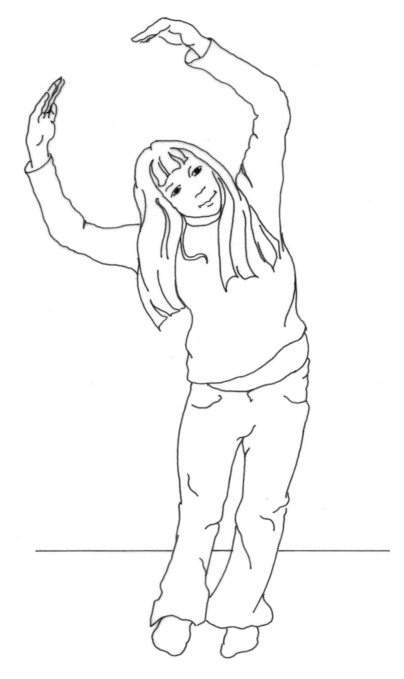

*Half moon (2)*

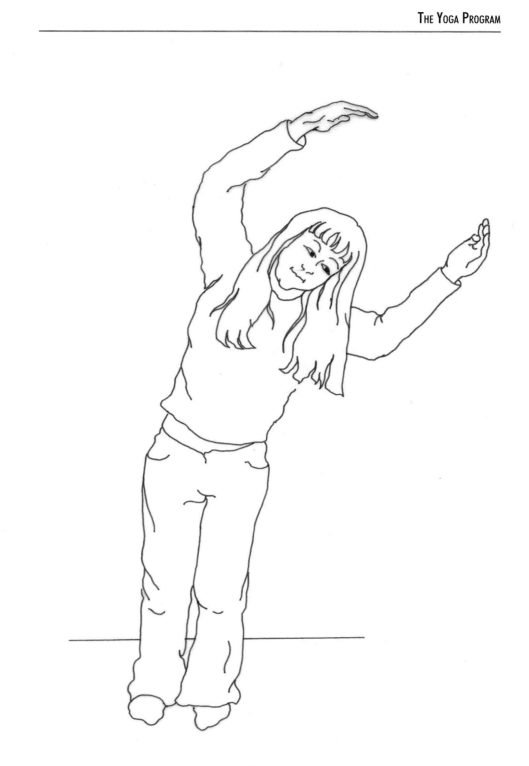

*Half moon (3)*

## HALF WHEEL

### *The posture*

Prepare yourself for Half Wheel by establishing Standing Mountain pose. To prepare, place your feet under your hips, tuck in your stomach, roll your shoulders back and down, and align your neck with your body. Inhale and move your arms upward over your head, with palms facing one another. Tighten your buttocks to protect your lower back, and gently lean backward, arching your body and keeping your arms long and extended.

### *The benefits*

This posture creates expansion and elongation of the chest. By tightening the buttocks you are teaching the child to protect his lower spinal vertebrae from stress. Some children may not align their head between their arms, and this can affect the flow of movement. Guide them to place their upper arms almost touching their ears.

### *Special considerations*

If a child demonstrates rounded shoulders I encourage her to stand tall and reach upward with both arms. If standing balance is an issue for a child, I often substitute this posture with an opportunity to lie gently back on a large therapy ball, in a straight-leg sitting position.

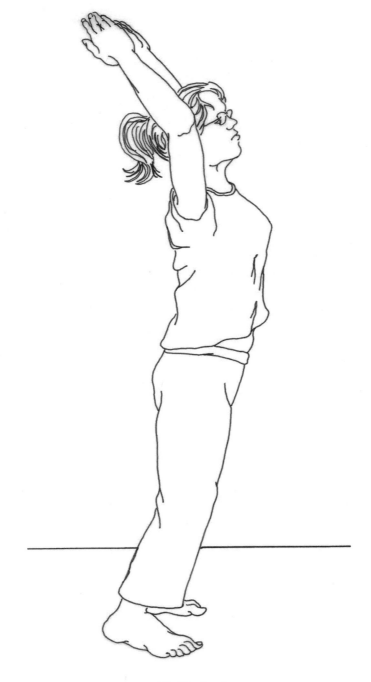

*Half wheel*

## UMBRELLA

### The posture

Standing with your feet placed across the width of the mat, and with your knees slightly bent, reach your arms behind you and lace your fingers together. Bend your body forward from the waist and raise your hands upwards, away from your back. Breathe in through your nose and gently out through your mouth. Lower your arms to your back and gently release your hands. Slowly roll up into standing, one vertebra at a time. Stand still and breathe.

### The benefits

Umbrella pose moves the shoulder blades over the back and externally rotates and stretches the shoulders. It is an inversion and allows the heart a rest from normal gravity posture while circulating more blood (and oxygen) to the upper body and head.

### Special considerations

A child may lock his knees or elbows to attempt to stabilize this posture. This locking can put undue stress on the knee joints. I am careful to encourage gentle bending at the knees and elbows to soften the stretch. If a child has any difficulty with shoulder joints, I do not do this pose and substitute the Rag Doll pose. Hanging in Rag Doll allows the arms to fall towards the mat as the body drops forward into an inversion.

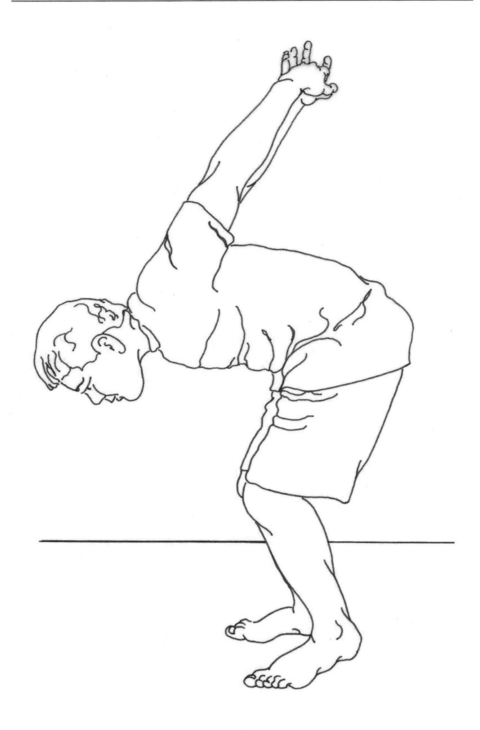

*Umbrella*

## TRIANGLE

### The posture

Place your feet three feet apart. Turn your right foot outward while pushing through your left heel. Inhale and move your arms up parallel to the surface of the mat, and exhale as you bend your body to the right and bring your fingertips down toward the floor. Do not bend forward, but sideways from the waist, keeping your legs straight. Your left arm is pointing toward the ceiling, forming a straight line with the right arm, which is pointing toward the mat. Inhale and move your body back into straight standing. Slowly exhale your arms down to your sides. Turn your right foot forward and your left foot outward. Push your right heel outward as you inhale your arms up parallel to the mat, and bend from your waist to the left. Your left fingers will be pointing toward the mat while your right arm is reaching straight to the ceiling. Legs are straight and your body is bent at the waist. Inhale, move your body back to standing as you exhale and move your arms down to your sides. Turn your left foot forward and gently jump, bringing your feet together.

### The benefits

Triangle provides a deep lateral stretch to the body. This posture is a balance pose with an inversion. The benefits of breathing through a lateral stretch encourage rib expansion as well as the opportunity for the circulatory system to replenish the upper body and brain.

### Special considerations

This posture varies in appearance, depending on the flexibility at the child's hip joints. It is important that the pose is a sideways rotating bend and that the child is not bending forward.

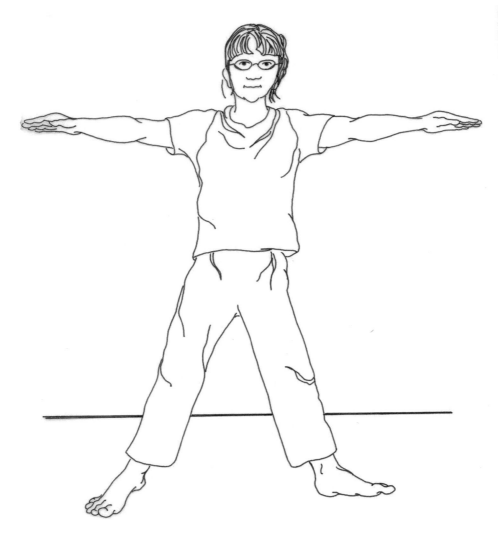

*Triangle (1)*

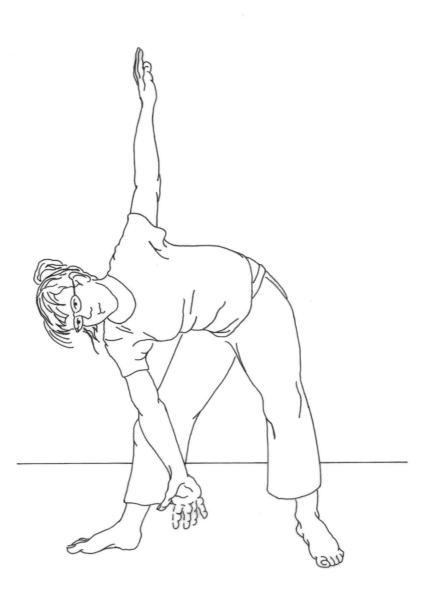

*Triangle (2)*

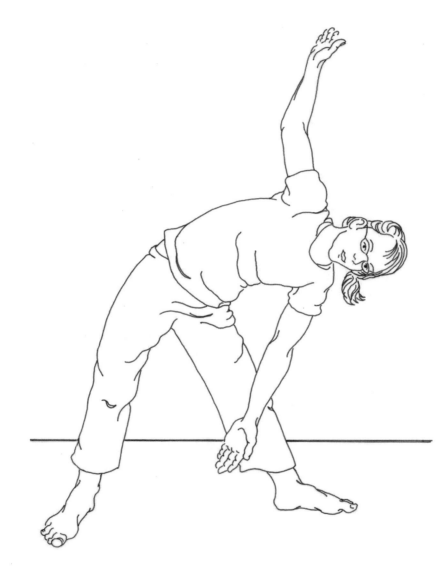

*Triangle (3)*

## TREE POSE

### The posture

Move into Standing Mountain pose. Stand on one leg and place the sole of your other foot on the inside of your standing leg. If it is difficult for you to place your foot above or below the knee of the standing leg, then place your foot on your ankle with the tip of your big toe still on the mat. Breathe and focus on one spot directly in front of you.

### The benefits

Tree pose is a standing balance pose that requires a visual focus and steady gaze to maintain balance. Rhythmic breathing supports the balance.

### Special considerations

Many children find Tree pose difficult. It may be necessary to have the child begin steady breathing and establish a visual focus before asking her to place the moving foot on the standing ankle. This pose seems to be particularly difficult for those children who have difficulty paying attention, and those who do not have a solid, flat foot base of support. If Tree pose is not possible for a child, due to structural or attention difficulties, I encourage them to maintain Standing Mountain pose.

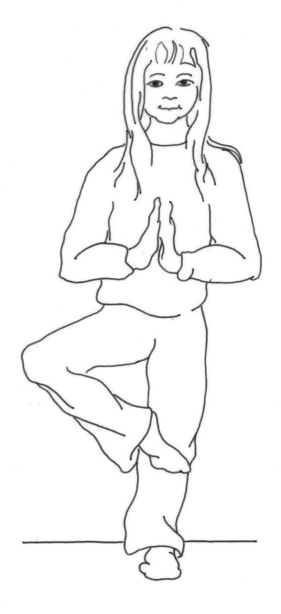

*Tree pose*

## HELICOPTER (REPEATED IN SEQUENCE OF POSES FOR REALIGNMENT OF SPINE)

*The posture*

First, move into Standing Mountain pose. Then, with arms hanging limp at your sides, begin to twist your body to the right, and then left. Let your arms swing around your body and even tap into your hips as you turn. Be sure that you are bending both knees, and when you turn to the right, be sure your left knee rotates to the right with your body. Do the same with a left twist and the right knee turning to the left with you. This protects the lower vertebrae, which do not rotate on a hinge.

*The benefits*

Helicopter realigns the spine, and at the same time provides vestibular stimulation. This posture is practiced spontaneously by some special needs children, and has been found to be a relaxing and reorienting experience for them. Helicopter further allows practice of maintaining balance while shifting weight from one foot to the other.

*Special considerations*

Children with low tone often begin this pose by fixing and remaining tight throughout the shoulder girdle and arms. Some children need to be reminded of the importance of bending the knees and following through with knee rotation on the twist. Explain this by providing an example they are familiar with, such as swinging a baseball bat.

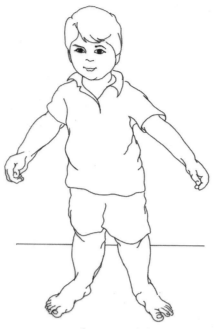

*Helicopter (1)*

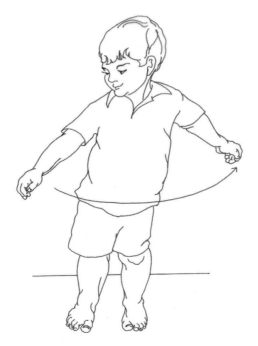

*Helicopter (2)*

## SAVASANA WITH GUIDED IMAGERY

*The posture*

Lie down on your back on the mat and rest your arms comfortably near your body, with your palms upward to receive. Lift your buttocks up and press your back into the mat. Place your eye bag over your eyes and relax. Let your body breathe you. Caution. Children with tactile sensitivity may find a mildly warm eye bag to be too much for their eyes. When heating eye bags use a 30 second limit and check the temperature of the bag by placing it over your eyes. Always hand the eye bag to your child and allow them to check the temperature before placing it over their eyes. If they need help with placement, be prepared to remove it quickly if they feel it is too warm. Take the time to determine the perfect microwave setting for your child.

*The benefits*

*Savasana* is the relaxing back lying pose that is used at the end of a yoga class in order to allow all parts of the body and mind to integrate the benefits of the entire yoga class. With increased oxygenation to the body the brainwaves may alter during a yoga class and produce a more meditative state by the end of the sequence. Within this altered state the mind more easily integrates information that is provided to the child.

This is the optimal window to introduce positive guided imagery. In this meditation state the brain perceives internal images in the same way as open-eyed stimuli. As the body-and-mind integration occurs, there is a state of balance within that creates improved inner harmony. This inner state of the child reflects a more true state of peacefulness, joy and love. Awareness is more sensitized and positive, and the child is more inwardly focused. Guided imagery stimulates a positive experience that is recorded deeply in the brain. Below is a guided imagery meditation that you can read to your child (or children) as they lie in this relaxed posture.

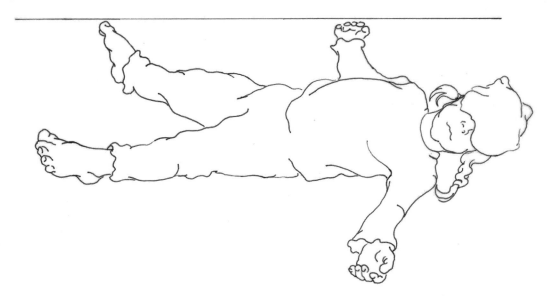

*Savasana with eyebag*

## Special considerations

If a child has difficulty lying still on the mat, a blanket can be tucked around her to provide proprioceptive input. If the eye bag overstimulates the child, remove it and tell the child to close her eyes. The eye bags that I use are designed with natural lavender and can be heated in a microwave to release the scent. The warmth generally comforts the child and helps her relax. Any eye bag will help the child by eliminating outer distraction.

Occasionally there is a child who cannot lie still and keep his eyes closed, and this is a perfect opportunity to supplement with Reiki. Reiki is a light, hands-on treatment that is based on sharing energy to calm, uplift and create a state of contentment. Gently place the palms of your hands on the top of the child's head, or over his eyes to help him calm. I guide the child through a few deep nasal inhalations and ask him to hold for the count of three before slowly exhaling. A restless child is then often able to calm and move into a deeper state of breathing.

## "Reflection in pool" meditation

Standing quietly on the top of a gently sloping grassy hill, you see a still pond sparkling in the sun below you. Walking slowly down the hill, your toes gripping the soft green grass, you stop at the edge of the water. Looking around, you see beautiful wild flowers in colors of red, orange and yellow. Taking a deep breath, you can smell the sweet scent of the flowers and the fragrance of grass that has been warmed by the sun. Bending your head, you look into the still pond and see that the reflection is as clear as a mirror.

Looking back at you is a long, sleek neck with smooth, wet feathers and a small, white head with a black beak. As you move closer to see white, feathered wings, the damp grass allows you to slide easily into the pond. You now float on a soft white belly, gliding so smoothly that it feels as if you are floating on the surface of the pond. With webbed feet you propel yourself through the water and understand that you are a graceful swan, gliding across a pool of green-blue water. [*Pause.*] Testing your ability to move in the water, you begin to swim in circles, around and around and around. As you move faster you realize that you are moving not by webbed feet any longer, but by a tail that is quickly flipping from side to side.

As you shoot from the water, creating a large spray, you know that you have become a fish. You no longer move with a soft glide, but with energetic spins and twists of your fins. [*Breathe deeply.*] Diving deep into the water, you see the sun reflect off the rocks on the bottom of the pond. Gaining speed, you burst through the surface of the water, bending from side to side until you feel the strong pull of air beneath what had been fins.

Now you see the flash of long, red wings that pull you higher over the pond. As you look down to the spot where you created ring upon ring of moving water patterns, your reflection shows you that you have changed into a beautiful red bird. Upward, moving through cooler and cooler air, you feel the freedom that only you are supporting by the rhythmic flapping of wings. [*Pause.*] Gliding above trees, grass and the sparkling pond, you see a reflection of the bird you have created. Wings reaching wide, feet tucked below your breast, you cruise towards a tall tree, where you gently land upon an upper branch. From this height you observe soft purple and pink clouds as the sun begins to set.

Moving slowly sideways, you observe that your claws now grip from between soft paws of fur. Your movement along the branch is slow and careful. Claws holding bark, arching your back, you move into a crouched position. From this tall perch you glance out across the grassy field, searching for any danger below. With keen vision and feline skill, you begin to move down the trunk of the tree, carefully, slowly. You are no ordinary cat, and have acquired the awareness of one who has lived among the trees and the animals. Lying low, hiding in the grass, you leap forward, prepared to pounce. Landing harder than you expected, you are aware of the sudden increase in your ability to smell your surroundings. [*Breathe deeply.*]

As you run eagerly, the sound of panting reaches your ears. The deep sensation in your throat results in wonderment as you hear yourself release a loud, strong bark. Jumping through the grass, you are pleased with the speed and strength with which you are able to propel yourself. This play has made you thirsty and you bound to the side of the pond to lower your head and lap up the water. The slurping of your puppy tongue changes into a sipping sound. There, staring back at you is the face you know so well.

Staring at the familiar eyes, you feel yourself come back into your body. Reaching a finger toward your reflection, you touch what you remember is you, sending ripples across the still water. Watching, you see the changes the ripples make as they move across your face. [*Pause.*] Smiling, you turn and walk slowly back up the grassy hill to where you came from. Feeling glad, you remember that you can visit this pond whenever you wish. By closing your eyes as you stand by the pond, you can become all the things you imagine yourself to be.

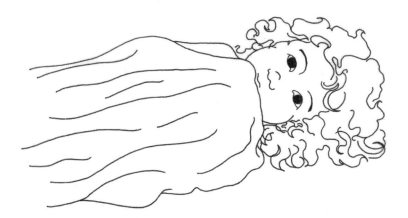

*Savasana with blanket*

## CLOSURE OF *SAVASANA*

### *The posture*

Begin to breathe more deeply now and come back into the room. Feel yourself lying on your yoga mat and gently wiggle your fingers and toes. Continue to breathe more deeply, and when you are ready, roll to one side and breathe there. Slowly push yourself up into sitting and keep your eyes closed.

### *The benefits*

A soft, slow transition is important when bringing a child back from a meditative state. Gentle and simple instructions are important in maintaining the calm and peaceful effect that *savasana* can provide. This transition allows the child to maintain the balance and calm that were established through the time of rest and integration. Guiding the child to keep his eyes closed can sustain inner awareness and preserve the calm state.

### *Special considerations*

A child who has gone deeply into a meditative state may need repeated encouragement to return to the room by soft calling of their name. It is preferable to use a soft voice to lead the child out of meditation. Touching him while he is in this state might be too abrupt and alerting.

Many children are not initially comfortable keeping their eyes closed in final mudra and mantra.

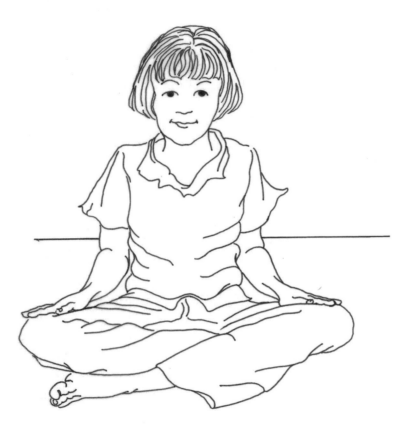

*Lotus*

## CLOSING MUDRA AND MANTRA

*The posture*

Please move into crossed legs sitting with your eyes closed. Form the OM mudra with both hands by making a circle with the thumb and index finger, and place your hands on your knees with your palms up. Sit tall and take a deep breath through your nose.

We will chant three OMs and two *shantis* the Sanskit term meaning peace, chanted to lift one's inner vibration into a balance of harmony. (Breathe through your nose audibly to cue the student to begin. Chant "OM" and repeat this two more times. Now chant *"shanti"* and repeat this one more time.) Place your hands in *namasté* and open your eyes slowly. I thank you for coming. *Namasté* [child's name]. (In a setting where it is you and your child, bow and say *"Namasté"* and have your child repeat this to you. In a group you address each child in turn, and await the child's reply.)

*The benefits*

The importance of the closing mantra and mudra is multifold. First, it allows the child to return slowly and gently to a more alert state. The chant, or mantra, allows the body to ground and balance itself. It also creates a harmonious connection among all present in the class. This harmony closes the session with the same intention as that with which it began: "All is one."

Having the eyes closed facilitates continuation of that inward state in which the connection with others is felt rather than observed. Visual distraction is eliminated and feeling is enhanced.

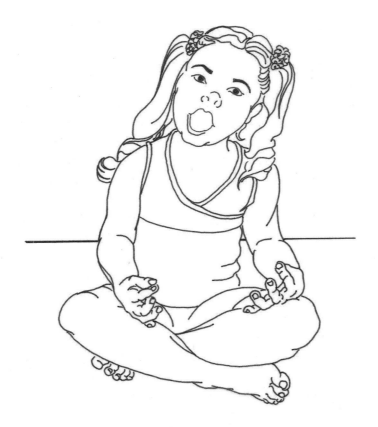

*Chanting and OM mudra*

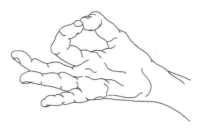

*OM mudra*

The OM mudra symbolizes the willingness to receive, as represented by the open and upward placement of the palms of the hands encouraging external rotation of the arms and wrists. The shape of this mudra reinforces a continuous circle of energy, represented in the shape formed by the thumb and index finger. Fine motor skills are encouraged by the fingertip formation. The connection between the gesture and the vocalized OM supports whole language for pre-verbal children.

## Special considerations

Hands placed palms up are perfect for a child who cannot form the delicate finger placement of the OM mudra. Any attempt to make contact with any finger is acceptable. If a child does not keep his eyes closed, he will be able to view the teacher with her eyes closed, and may eventually imitate.

In a yoga protocol each pose is carefully selected not only to deliver stretch, elongation and strengthening to the physical body, but also to stimulate the "energy body." Each pose stimulates one or more of seven main energy centers in the body. These energy centers, called charkas, are situated along the spine, with the first chakra revolving around the coccyx or base of the spine, and the seventh chakra spinning at the top of the head. The importance of these energy chakras will be explained in the next chapter.

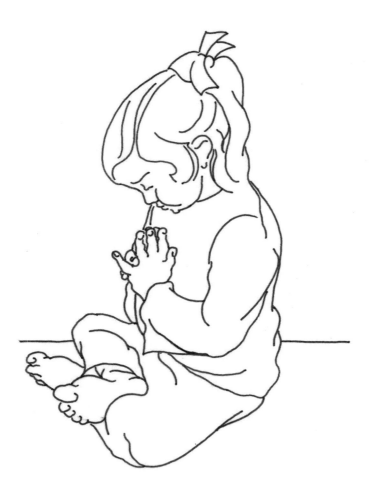

*Namasté*

# 5

## YOGA AND THE ENERGY BODY

So far in this book, the benefits of yoga therapy for the physical/structural body have been reviewed, with attention given to special considerations. Yoga therapy is also beautiful for a second body, however—one that is invisible to the eye, but felt within—what is known in yoga as the energy body. When our energy body is balanced, it comfortably aligns with the physical body to create a feeling of wholeness and health. Many people refer to this as "the yoga zone" or state of bliss. When the energetic body is not balanced we can experience a sense of irritation, anxiety or lack of balance. When you feel the beautiful space of peace and calm in a yoga class, this indicates that the physical and energetic bodies are balanced and working together.

In this invisible body, there are seven primary centers of energy housed along the spine. They start at the tail bone and end at the top of the head. These major energy centers are called chakras. Each chakra area stores energy that stimulates lessons that support our journey to become the best that we can be. These energies influence how we view our world, love ourselves and others and develop the ability to make wise choices in our life. It is important to understand these centers because yoga stimulates the energetic body and awakens the lessons that are stored within them. Each yoga pose stimulates one or more energy centers, and the yoga therapy sequence has been carefully designed to move energy effectively through the body for a full balancing. The child who participates in this specially designed sequence improves a vast array of physical skills and also awakens to the awareness of values and choices in everyday lessons of life. For a child with special needs, life's journey can sometimes be a bit rough, and a program that guides him in self-awareness and development can be a precious gift.

## THE ROOT CHAKRA—STABILITY

The first lesson stored within the energetic body is about establishing our foundation. This energy is located in the root chakra at the base of our tail bone, and where our body contacts the earth when sitting. This area stores lessons around the ways in which we connect with the world, such as through family, home, roots, for security and survival. Before we can grow, we must first have a solid footing in the world and learn to understand the oneness of family and community. The child is learning about group identity and how he fits within the group.

It is important for children to know the security of their family unit and thrive through connection in their world. Feeling secure at home builds the foundation for the child to gain the confidence that he or she needs to individuate and explore outside the immediate family.

In addition to love and acceptance there are many activities to help a child understand the importance of being grounded.

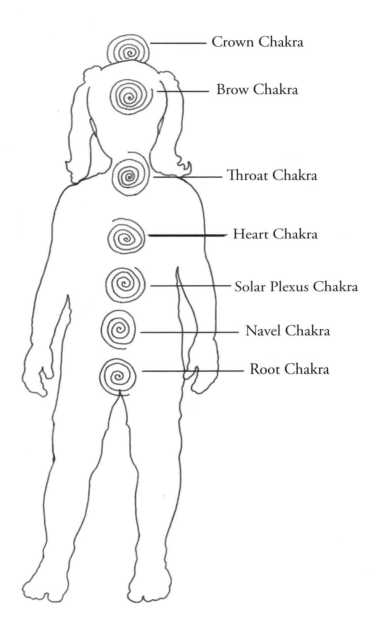

Crown Chakra

Brow Chakra

Throat Chakra

Heart Chakra

Solar Plexus Chakra

Navel Chakra

Root Chakra

*Positions of the Chakras*

*Yoga focus*

- Leg extensions: see pages 54—57.

- Forward bend: see pages 66—67.

- Sway pose: see pages 88—91.

- Squat: see pages 100—101.

ADDITIONAL ACTIVITIES

- Love to the Planet: see page 151.

- Being a Tree: see page 154.

## THE NAVEL CHAKRA—RELATIONSHIP AND CREATIVITY

Moving upward along the spine to the abdominal area, we find the location of the next energy center. When this area of the body is stimulated with yoga we become more aware of lessons about relating to others, and also begin the process of individuating from the family or tribe. The child begins to form friendships outside the immediate family. The understanding of healthy parameters is forming, along with the rhythm of giving and receiving.

A yoga environment naturally supports harmonious relationship with self, which can provide more confidence in relating to others. Opening each yoga therapy session with *namasté* creates an environment of honor and respect. The atmosphere is soft, quiet, visually uncluttered, and calm music is playing as the child enters the yoga area. The intention is for the peaceful environment to mirror the inner world. The stage has been set for calm and peaceful cooperation. The child's yoga mat defines her personal space and supports her understanding of personal boundaries.

Another lesson in this energy center is about developing creative expression with others. As outlined in the next chapter, there is a wealth of opportunities to creatively interact within a therapeutic yoga session. Below are some suggestions for practices in which children learn to create together. If you are working in a one-to-one setting, partner up with your child. If you are working with a small group, divide the children into pairs.

## Yoga focus

- Yoga mudra: see pages 48—49.
- Spinal twist: see pages 58—61.
- Arch: see pages 62—63.
- Helicopter: see pages 104—105.
- Triangle: see pages 114—117.

ADDITIONAL ACTIVITIES

- Teacher: see page 150.
- Breathing partners: see page 153.
- Continuous story: see page 156.

## THE SOLAR PLEXUS CHAKRA—SELF-ESTEEM

The energy center located above our waist and below our heart is the center for personal power and self-esteem. This is the center where the child's identity is cultivated and energy is exchanged between the child and the environment. The lessons stimulated in this area of the body support the child's development of a sense of purpose and the establishment of self-control. With the cultivation of self-control the child begins to learn how to slow down and begin accepting responsibility for the type of person he is to become. Transmuting anger and fear are important parts of these lessons.

The child with special needs often has obstacles that make it more challenging to achieve goals and cultivate the self-esteem that accompanies those achievements. Yoga is a setting where each person is perfect as they are, and the difference between one person and the next is simply an observation of how unique we are. Yoga comprises a wealth of techniques that stimulate various systems in the body and can help the child work through challenges and improve her ability to succeed.

Many of the children in therapeutic yoga have learned yoga technique in class and have been able to carry these skills effectively into other environments. Several students have explained that they stop and do their yoga breathing when they become anxious or upset. Other children have told me they are able to remember to respect others by taking turns or listening to their needs. The ability to carry over the yoga calm into each and every environment is a skill that can be mastered in a yoga practice.

## Yoga focus

- Arch: see pages 62—63.
- Spinal roll: see pages 64—65.
- Cat: see pages 92—93.
- Half Wheel: see pages 110—111.

ADDITIONAL ACTIVITIES

- Guided imagery: see pages 122—128.
- Positive affirmations: see page 148.

## THE HEART CHAKRA—LOVE AND COMPASSION

The heart chakra is located in the middle of the chest, close to the physical heart. Here we learn the lessons of love, compassion and how to heal past wounds. This energy center marks the midway point in the body's seven primary chakras: the heart center operates between the three lower centers that pertain primarily to the lessons of the outside world and the three upper chakras that are related to lessons of our inner world.

In the heart chakra, we learn about the qualities of loving and being loved. There are lessons of openness, giving, receiving, balance and compassion. This center is involved in our impressions of self-acceptance. When we accept and love ourselves, it is much easier to share love and accept others. Within our heart chakra is stored our emotional power, and also our ability to forgive. The children enjoy all activities that involve loving self and others. The practices described below are designed to open the heart and promote a loving feeling within.

## Yoga focus

- Spinal twist: see pages 58—61.

- Volcano: see pages 70—73.

- Child's Pose: see pages 98—99.

ADDITIONAL ACTIVITIES

- Heart Mudra: see page 147.

- Love to the Planet: see page 151.

## THE THROAT CHAKRA—COMMUNICATION

We move up to the fifth energy center, located in the throat. When this center is stimulated in a yoga pose, lessons of self-expression arise. In addition, skills pertaining to rhythm, sound, connection, singing, chanting, writing and public speaking are in focus. Here we learn the right to speak and to be heard. It is always our goal to be clear in our communications, and when this chakra is balanced, we are more able to reach that goal.

For children with a speech/language delay or disorder there are additional challenges in discovering a way to be effectively understood. This can create stress and barriers in the give-and-take of expressing wants, needs and thoughts. When a child is limited in verbal expression, it is often more difficult for him to connect, be socially engaging and fulfill his needs of interacting with others. Yoga chanting, use of hand postures and motor planning of sequenced poses all support precursors to effective spoken communication.

Creative expression is exercised in the lessons of the throat charka, to include speaking, writing and artistic expression. Music and art may be motivating outlets for the child to explore. Expressive dance, painting and singing all constitute opportunities to exercise variety in expression and help to facilitate speech or written language skills. Chanting and breathing activities are also excellent choices in working with the energy of the throat chakra.

## Yoga focus

- Arch: see pages 62—63.

- Spinal roll: see pages 64—65.

- Upward-facing Dog: see pages 96—97.

ADDITIONAL ACTIVITIES

- Sipping breath: see page 152.

- Oyster breath: see page 153.

- Mudra and mantra games: see pages 147—148.

## THE BROW CHAKRA—DIVINE VISION

Our sixth chakra or energy center is located in the brow area. It is often referred to as our "third eye." Imagination and intuition are stimulated in this center, and self-reflection is evoked. Awakening to the soul, as well as concentration, wisdom, insight and peace of mind are all lessons located in the brow center. Other aspects of this area include dreams, beauty, vision and color.

Guided imagery stimulates the lessons of the sixth chakra. Once a child becomes balanced by participating in the yoga postures of the program, it is time to encourage visual creation by means of guided imagery. This is how imagination is cultivated, and the potential of thought expands. Children have had less time on the planet than adults to formulate mental limitations, and they are still open to creating their dreams. I have observed many children move their arms in flight on their yoga mat when the guided imagery focused on a bird. It is not uncommon to see a child move her arm when you ask her to reach out and touch something in her visualization activity.

There is ample opportunity to be creative throughout the entire yoga session. Here are some practices that can stimulate the third eye energy of divine vision. Many more creative ideas are outlined in Chapter Six.

*Yoga focus*

- *Savasana*: see pages 50—51.
- Child's pose: see pages 98—99.

ADDITIONAL ACTIVITIES

- Decorate your Tree: see page 155.

## THE CROWN CHAKRA—SPIRITUAL CONNECTION

The crown charka is located at the top of the head. This energetic spot pertains to connection, grace, soul and the Universe. It is here that we feel the energy of self-unification, or a coming together of our personality with our highest self. Even very young children are aware of something greater than themselves and are interested in being their best.

The crown chakra is associated with inspiration and our relationship with that which is divine. It puts us in touch with our divine purpose and selfless service, and it teaches us to be present in the moment—something children typically express with ease. It holds our discovery of the knowledge that we are connected to all that is.

### Yoga focus

- *Savasana*: see pages 50—51.
- Guided Imagery: see pages 122—128.

ADDITIONAL ACTIVITIES

- Circular OM: see page 147.

# 6

## YOGA GAMES

Playful embellishments to the yoga program add fun and a creative spirit and do not alter the importance of the original sequence.

This chapter describes creative games that support the benefits of the yoga program and provide you with choices for stimulating a specific skill. You may wish to try out a yoga game when you have time for just one activity. Alternatively, a game can be an excellent way to begin a session or to transition from breathing exercises into mudra and mantra at the beginning of the yoga program. Offering your child a choice of two different games encourages their participation in the design of the session. Enjoy! This is meant to be fun.

## GAMES TO BUILD STRENGTH

Maintaining a pose, for example, Downward dog, for a longer period of time is a good way of building strength. Another way to accomplish this is by moving in weight bearing poses such as Table or Cat pose. Alternatively, you might try some of these fun games.

### Crab in the ocean

One activity that builds strength through weight bearing is moving in crab walk. First, move into Crab pose by sitting with your knees bent and your arms and hands behind you supporting your weight. Lift your buttocks up off the sand and push your stomach towards the sky. Walk on your hands and feet like a crab as you move and walk towards the ocean. Next, when the ocean tide comes onto the beach, the crab scurries backwards to stay dry. As the child repeats alternately walking forwards and scurrying backwards, he is building strength in his legs, arms and trunk.

### Jumping frogs

Squat pose has been referred to by many names, but one of the most common is Frog pose. The children transition into Squat pose and then hop gently on their mats. Yes, of course the children "ribbet"!

### Flamingo walk

Another favorite yoga game is posing as a flamingo. When standing in Tree pose (with one leg bearing all of your weight and the other knee bent, with the foot on your extended leg) you resemble a flamingo. To play this game you walk behind the teacher, but when she stops and turns around to look, you must be standing in flamingo pose. If a child has been caught not posing in flamingo, they must go back five steps. The first child to make it as far as the teacher wins the game. Not only is there movement, strengthening and balance, but speed and rhythm are crucial to succeed in this game.

## MUDRA AND MANTRA GAMES

Mudra and mantra games are fun, offer a means of communication for nonverbal children, and are a good way to encourage sequenced motor planning. Here are some activities to add to those you have learned in the yoga program.

### Heart mudra

Form the OM mudra with both hands by making a circle with the thumb and index finger. Let the other three fingers fan away from the palm of your hand. Bring the long middle fingers of each hand together, tip to tip. Now place the circular ring of your thumb and index finger of the *right* hand, on your heart. Breathe.

### Circular OM

Singing OM in a round is an excellent game to practice the timing of starting and stopping. If you are working with one child, take turns at beginning and finishing the OM chant. If you are working in a small group, have each child chant OM in turn, beginning when you point to them. When you point to him again, the child stops, then begins the chant once more.

### Hari OM

Hari OM is sung by clapping to the beat of each syllable in the lyrics of the song. The lyrics are Hari OM, Hari OM, OM, OM, OM. Your child imitates you clapping two beats as you lean your body to the right and sing Hari OM, followed by two beats as you lean your body to the left and sing Hari OM. Raising your hands high above you clap three consecutive times as you sing the final syllables OM, OM, OM.

147

As you sing the song "Hari OM" call out the word that will be paired with OM in the next repeat. The leader of the song points to a child, who will then call out the word for the next repeat. The timing is important, so that the continuity and rhythm of the song is not delayed. The vocabulary choices consist of:

- Hari OM

- Shanti OM

- Shiva OM.

## GAMES TO BUILD CONFIDENCE

In the special needs population, I frequently observe hesitancy about initiating an activity or acting as a leader. There is often a lack of self confidence and a fear of standing out. Often the child develops into a skilled leader with ample technique for effectively teaching another.

### Positive affirmations

Repeating positive statements can train the mind to focus on what is positive, allowing any negative thoughts to fall away. Claiming the beauty within you is uplifting and supportive. Children can repeat these affirmations following guided imagery, and in this way more deeply integrate the positive effects.

- I am peace.

- I am love.

- I am joy.

- I am light.

- I shine with my inner light.

- I dance with joy.

## "Yogi Says"

In this activity the rules for "Simon Says" are used to encourage awareness of detailed directions. You start by asking the child to do certain poses. If preceded with "Yogi Says" the pose is to be performed. If the directions are not preceded by "Yogi Says" the pose is not to be performed. When a child performs a pose without the necessary "Yogi Says" they then become the teacher. This is an excellent way to teach finer listening skills and also to support expressive language skills. The ultimate purpose of the game, however, is to encourage leadership skills and a sense of confidence.

## Guided imagery

I teach yoga therapy to two children diagnosed with Asperger syndrome who love to lead guided imagery. This is an opportunity for the children to use their creativity and demonstrate responsibility for guiding another person into a quiet place. I have observed success when a child has led the guided imagery, both in a one-to-one setting and in small groups.

## Tibetan bells

The Tibetan bells are passed to the child and he takes a turn ringing them. This is a simple skill that allows him to begin a leadership role by demonstration rather than complex spoken directions.

## Sharing

A sharing often takes place following guided imagery. Some children wish to elaborate on their experiences and describe in detail what they saw.

## Teacher

There are many opportunities in yoga for the child to take on the role of teacher. Whether it is leading a breathing activity or teaching a pose, they take responsibility for guiding the teacher. This is an excellent opportunity for them to express their understanding of the details of a pose and to use their language concepts of position, directionality and quality.

## GAMES USING PROPS AND TOYS

Over time I have added tangible items to the sequence and found that glitter balls, sashes, simple instruments, finger puppets and bubbles can provide motivation when teaching yoga to children.

## Glitter balls

Not only are these balls beautiful to look at, they are also fun to incorporate into the basic sequence. Each child chooses the color of their ball and is then asked to follow the teacher in working with it. The ball is passed from hand to hand, overhead, behind the back, and in Butterfly breathing. During Butterfly pose the child places the ball on top of his feet and maintains it there during the transition into Flower pose.

Children seem to demonstrate a more artistic flow with their poses when the ball is added to the program. They are more careful and flowing with their movements when they become the backdrop for the ball.

## Sashes

Sashes are often used in yoga to extend a stretch or facilitate a bend. I use colorful Guatemalan sashes that I have found at import stores. This material is easier for little hands to hold than the traditional canvas straps used in yoga. Use straps to deepen the stretch in Umbrella, forward bend and in straight leg stretches.

Using straps makes the child more aware of the stretch, and gives her practice in using a tool to improve her yoga pose.

## Musical instruments

In yoga gatherings for mantra, chanting and mudra (sequenced hand postures), instruments are often used to expand the experience. In yoga therapy, hand-held maracas and simple bells let the children add another modality to their participation, and allow for fine motor activity and creative self-expression. For a child who is having difficulty with the actual verbal production of mantra, this is an opportunity to communicate with gestures.

## Love to the planet

One of the favorite activities in yoga therapy is "sending love to the planet". The child sits in front of a flat, atlas board map and places a rose quartz gemstone, cut into a heart shape, or any symbol of love, on the location to which he wishes to send love. It is beautiful to watch a child place his gemstone and send his love to a country he feels would benefit from his highest regard. This activity broadens one's family to include the world and view the people across the planet as brothers and sisters. Having a physical object to place on the map and a visual representation of the entire planet makes the process seem more real. It helps the child see (literally) that we all share the same planet.

## Whistles, bells and bubbles

The simple plastic whistle designed like a straw is often used in yoga therapy as a tool to demonstrate finer grading of breath. The child is asked to blow the whistle, but to do it softly. The feedback from the whistle helps guide the child to stronger or softer breath flow.

Bubbles are also used to teach deeper inhalations and longer, more even exhalations. When the child makes the desired exhalation, it will result in a large bubble. Less even blowing results in smaller bubbles. It is helpful to demonstrate the softness by exhaling your breath onto the child's hand. The child will feel how softly the breath is released.

The Tibetan bells can also be used to demonstrate smooth movement: when the child brings the bells together with skill, the sound is softer.

## BREATHING GAMES

Breathing is a natural function that we typically take for granted. When we learn to focus on our breath, we become more aware of how breathing more deeply and evenly can improve how we feel, talk, exercise and eat. Children also need to bring focus to the breath and learn to carry it over into their daily lives to improve a variety of activities. There are many breathing techniques in yoga that become more fun with a touch of added creativity.

### Sipping breath

Sitting with your legs together and straight in front of you, fold over into a forward bend. Next, slowly move up into straight sitting while sipping air into your mouth. "Sipping breath" is characterized by sucking in several small breaths as you move upwards. During this breathing technique I have the children describe which thick beverage they are sipping through their straw. Smoothies and milkshakes are favorites for many of the children.

## Oyster breath

Using a sipping breath technique as described above, and with an imaginary pearl resting in your lap, you can imagine you are an oyster closing forward to protect your pearl. This image frequently facilitates a deeper stretch.

## Bellows breath

Bellows breathing is characterized by breathing in and out of the nose with your body acting much like a bellows. The body moves more upright with each inhalation, and relaxes downward with each exhalation.

Once this breathing activity has been mastered, variations in speed can be used to achieve what we call "choo-choo breathing." Begin bellows breathing very slowly, and progressively speed up the inhalations and exhalations until your nasal breathing sounds like a train moving down the railroad track.

## Breathing partners

Take turns with the child, as one person blows the bubbles and the other returns them. At the beginning of a yoga class, children in a group setting share the bubble-blowing breathing activity with a partner. Turn-taking is necessary, and it is up to the partners to determine when to swap roles.

## Three-part breathing

In the practice of three-part breathing you visualize the breath, first filling your chest just below the neck, next filling the heart spot, and finally filling the stomach area. During exhalation feel the breath leaving first, the stomach area, next, the heart area, and last, the upper chest area.

This flow of inhalation and exhalation is similar to the effect of a balloon being fully inflated and then slowly releasing the air until it is empty. Guide the child through the slow inhalation steps, describing a balloon becoming larger and larger as it fills. Describe the air leaving the balloon, how it thins and becomes empty.

## Healing breath

Lying on your back, begin to breathe deeply into your body. The next breath you take will go wherever you want it to go in your body: see the breath move through you and into that exact spot. Watch the breath circle around that specific part of your body. Take the next breath to this same spot, or to another spot. Again, watch the breath circle that part of your body. Now feel the breath take away any pain you are feeling in that spot. Continue to breathe wherever you want to feel better, seeing the breath circle and hug that spot. What you see in your head can become real.

## GAMES TO DEVELOP IMAGINATION

### Being a tree

Stand up and place your feet slightly apart. Imagine the floor as soft, dark earth and your legs as a tree trunk. Feel roots growing from the soles of your feet and beginning to burrow into the earth. Feel the roots you have sprouted slowly moving further down into the soil and securing you in one spot. Now raise your arms above your head and move them in the way you would see tree branches gently blowing in the wind. The more you allow your roots to grow and support you, the higher and wider your branches grow. Feel how comfortable it is to know you have roots to hold you in place, and how uplifted you are with branches and blossoms growing from your trunk.

## Decorate your tree

We used "Being a tree" as an activity for the first chakra (see page 138). In the activities for the base chakra we had the child be a tree. Decorating that tree is a focus for the sixth chakra. Here the imagination is free to design and create whatever is colorful, beautiful, and from the place of dreams within the child. Teach the following:

Close your eyes and take a deep breath. Relax your body and take another breath. I want you to see yourself as a tree. You might be a pine tree with needles on your branches, or a large oak tree towering high in the sky. See your trunk, branches, needles or leaves, and the sky around and above you. Feel your roots securing you into the ground and your branches reaching for the sun.

You are going to decorate your tree and create what you think is beautiful. If you wish to have blossoms on your tree, see them there now. What shape are they, what color? You may want to grow fruit or pods on your tree. Are there any animals gracing your branches? Maybe there is a chipmunk or squirrel hiding nuts in a hole in your trunk, or a bird building a nest deep in your leafy branches.

There are so many ways to make your tree just as you wish it to be. Have you ever wanted a tree house with all of your favorite things inside of it? Maybe you would like to have a bird house and feeder in your tree. Hummingbirds like sugar water, and you could hang a feeder for them on one of your branches. A caterpillar just might spin his cocoon on one of your limbs, or maybe several butterflies will hatch from their chrysalises and fly around in a burst of color.

Take some time now to finish your tree and see it as you would like it to be. This is your tree and your creation, enjoy it now. Begin to breathe more deeply and remember that you can visit your tree any time you wish. All that you need to do is close your eyes and see yourself there, standing by your tree.

## Continuous story

In this activity a story is told as the children maintain the yoga pose that relates to the story. In Butterfly pose one child begins a story of where the butterfly is traveling, and the next person continues where the child left off. The children have the opportunity to share creativity while cooperating in a task. In a one-to-one setting, a parent and child can take turns, sharing a pose with a piece of the story. In a small group, everyone takes a turn.

## SONGS

Most children love music, and singing is one form of calming and uplifting. There are many familiar children's songs that speak of positive and joyful feelings. The movements of the "Hoky Poky" and "If You're Happy and You Know It" can be used as warm-up stretches when you move through the actions described in the lyrics.

I designed an eighteen minute music yoga CD titled "Songs to Grow On." Music often captures and maintains the attention of children and when using this CD I observed improved particpation from children ages two to fours years old.

# 7

## YOGA FOR SPECIFIC CONDITIONS

Through the observation and acceptance of our differences, we recognize that we are all one and the same. By using our strengths we are able to facilitate improvement in the areas of our life that are not yet balanced or integrated. There is always space for improvement, through our physical changes and/or our shifts in responsibility, beliefs and attitude. It is important to get to know our strengths and to use them to create a better quality of life in those areas that we have yet to master.

## PRECAUTIONS

No two children diagnosed with special needs reveal identical symptoms, nor does one child mirror another with the same symptoms. This is the beauty of the unique human being, and the miracle of our unique expression. Prior to placing a child into the yoga class and embarking on the gentle yoga sequence, it is imperative to review whichever of the following sections applies and adapt the program according to the alternatives that I have recommended.

The beauty of the yoga therapy sequence that I have presented is that it does not include advanced poses, and it has been planned with basic precautions in mind. Taking the basic sequence, with yoga games you should be able to develop a beautiful practice of yoga for your child. Using the information that pertains to the child's particular diagnosis and symptoms, you will be equipped to move forward with a safe, gentle and effective yoga program.

## ATTENTION DEFICIT/HYPERACTIVITY DISORDER (ADHD)

One of the natural beauties of yoga practice is the simple, calm environment that is essentially free of visual, auditory and tactile distractions. The yoga mat defines an area of personal space for the child. Music selected for class is designed to facilitate the qualities of inner calm and harmony, while natural lighting softens the environment. Once the child is completely familiar with the yoga program and comfortable with the yoga room, there is the potential to practice with eyes closed. At this level the child attends inwardly and is not affected by visual stimuli.

In a study by Haffner *et al.* (2006) where a comparison was made between the effectiveness of yoga for children and conventional motor exercise in a randomized controlled pilot study of children with ADHD. The outcome of this study revealed that the yoga training was superior to the conventional motor training. The authors found that over the course of the study all symptoms were reduced. Yoga was also reported to be particularly effective for those children receiving medication for ADHD. The researchers concluded that yoga can be an effective activity for improving performance of children diagnosed with ADHD.

Focused breathing relaxes and calms a child, and may contribute to changed brainwaves, all of which can help towards a reduced activity level. A reduction in movement may be observed in those children who are typically overactive. There is also an increase in focus when practicing conscious breathing exercises.

*Exchanges/deletions:*

None.

*Yoga focus for ADHD*

- Yoga breathing activities: see breathing games on pages 152–154 and Mudra and Mantra games on pages 147–148.

- Full yoga pose sequence: see Chapter Four.

## AUTISM SPECTRUM DISORDER (ASD)

The wide spectrum of symptoms found in autism can be as diverse as the benefits of yoga. A child with a diagnosis of autism can benefit from yoga, regardless of where they are diagnosed on the spectrum. Yoga can provide the comfort of a minimally distracting and familiar room, a designated mat from which to participate and a consistently familiar protocol. For a child with autism, who can be frightened by new surroundings, this simple venue, free of distractions, can become a secure arena in which to imitate and learn. A child with these characteristics responds well to one-on-one yoga therapy with an opportunity to work directly next to the therapist, be that the parent, teacher, or whoever else might be teaching the yoga program. Through the experience of repeated sequences, the child becomes comfortable with what is expected in the yoga therapy setting.

Many children with autism communicate through body posture, gesture, vocalizations and approximations of sign language. Yoga therapy meets the child at his level through the gross motor imitation of poses, the finer motor imitation of mudras and the vocal/verbal stimulation of mantras.

At the other end of the autism spectrum is the opportunity for a yoga therapy program to stimulate the curiosity and creative quest of children diagnosed with Asperger syndrome. Of paramount benefit is the opportunity to socialize with others, either in a one-on-one setting or, if a peer is able to practice yoga, with them. The context of respect set in a yoga therapy session helps to honor the reciprocity required for effective communication skills. Grading of voice and movement can facilitate calmer interactions and improve the likelihood of successful exchanges. Turn-taking prohibits extended self-focus from the child and makes it important to listen. Leadership skills are cultivated if the child agrees to teach a portion of the class.

In their book *Yoga for Children with Autism Spectrum Disorders*, authors Dion and Stacey Betts (2006) share the yoga program they used with their son Joshua. They found that yoga helped their son relieve the tension and anxiety that is often magnified in children diagnosed with Asperger syndrome.

Of particular interest to children who are diagnosed with Asperger syndrome are the creative and imaginative opportunities in yoga. The chance to expand on an activity is often met as a stimulating challenge, particularly if the expansion involves imagination. Mudra sequences, stories and detailed elaboration of existing poses are all of interest. I have worked with two children with ASD who love to lead guided imagery and they have both done an exceptional job.

*Exchanges/deletions*
    None

## *Yoga focus for autism*

- Mudra and mantra games: see pages 147–148.

- Breathing games: see pages 152–154.

- Full yoga pose sequence: see Chapter Four.

## *Yoga focus for Asperger syndrome*

- Games to develop imagination: see pages 154–156.

- Mudra and mantra games: see pages 147–148.

- Games using props and toys: see pages 150–151.

- Breathing games: see pages 152–154.

## CANCER

Many have reported the relaxing quality of yoga, and there is no doubt that deeper breathing helps us to cope with many varieties of stress in our lives. Fear and stress related to a serious or terminal illness can impact on our breathing, and it is important to be aware of breathing patterns where the inhalation/exhalation cycle is shallow, rapid or both.

Therapy services in the Seattle Cancer Care Unit inpatient care unit at the Children's Hospital Medical Center in Seattle, Washington, include a wide variety of activities, including, yoga therapy. The therapists seek to teach skills that can be practiced in daily life and support continued healthful growth and development.

## *Exchanges/deletions*

Consult the child's physician prior to initiating a yoga practice that includes postures.

*Yoga focus for cancer*

- Healing breath: see page 154.

- *Savasana*: see pages 50–51.

- Mudra and mantra games: see pages 147–148.

## CEREBRAL PALSY (CP)

As explained in Chapter One, yoga mirrors the work of the Bobaths' therapeutic intervention, neuro-developmental therapy (see page 14). In this treatment, children diagnosed with cerebral palsy are treated by emulating the developmental stages that a child would normally experience independently. The children are facilitated hand over hand up through gravity in the transitions of flexion, extension and rotation as they mirror a child's progression through normal gross and fine motor skills. The postures used in NDT mimic those of normal development as well as the progression from supine to standing used in a yoga class.

The opportunity to stretch and also build strength through yoga practice meets the complex needs of a child with CP. The addition of respiratory work enhances the opportunity for the child to bring more oxygen into a tight body. Respiration work in yoga is exactly the focus needed for children with CP, who often use compensatory patterns of pushing with extension to breathe. A more neutral position to retrain, improve and support breathing is automatically practiced in yoga.

Underneath the high tone of a child diagnosed with CP, there is often a low base of tone. For these children it is crucial to have opportunities to build strength by bearing weight. A therapeutic program that meets both low tone and high tone needs in one session while incorporating games, is extremely beneficial to a child diagnosed with CP. The addition of respiratory work seems custom-made for this population. Yoga meets all of those needs.

## Exchanges/deletions

Assist the child in any poses where he is unable to maintain balance. If the child is not standing independently, help him to come up onto his feet and support him around the trunk with his feet stabilized properly. Gently move the child in Helicopter pose.

## Yoga focus for cerebral palsy

- Full body stretch: see pages 52–53.

- Spinal twist: see pages 58–61.

- Leg extensions: see pages 54–57.

- Downward dog pose: see pages 94–95.

- Breathing games: see pages 152–154.

## COMPROMISED RESPIRATION

One of the keys to unlocking tightness and constrictions in part of the body is focused breathing during a yoga pose. Targeted deep breathing relaxes and oxygenates the body and exercises the respiratory muscles. The child learns the optimal coordination of the breathing cycle as he moves the various parts of his body. Yoga opens up the constricted portion of the body by stretching, and the next inhalation provides the oxygen to fill this previously constricted space.

Constant reminders to breathe retrain children who need to master deeper breathing habits. Breathing through the nose gives them greater control of inhalation and exhalation. When an exhalation has been released slowly and completely, the body automatically inhales more deeply. Yoga also teaches us not to hold our breath. Elevated arm poses challenge breathing and force us to take deeper inhalations.

A study by Cooper *et al.* (2003) revealed that Buteyko, a yoga breathing technique, improved symptoms and resulted in reduced use of a bronchodilator for a population of asthma patients.

### Exchanges/deletions

A physician's prescription is recommended for patients who have compromised respiration. Limit arms-over-head positions to one deep breath cycle.

### Yoga focus for compromised respiration

- Breathing games: see chest-expanding poses—Umbrella (pages 112–113), Butterfly Breathing (pages 74–78) and Half Wheel (pages 110–111).

- Rotation poses: see sitting spinal twist (pages 84–87) and Helicopter (pages 104–105).

- Extended arm poses: see Half Moon (pages 106–109), Volcano (pages 70–73) and sitting sway pose (pages 88–91).

## DEVELOPMENTAL DELAY

The outlined yoga sequence flows in a "developmental" model, from lying down, moving up against gravity through various positions and transitions into standing. The entire yoga therapy sequence supports and facilitates flexion, extension and rotation following the order of normal developmental postures and transitions.

Yoga therapy addresses all developmental skill areas, including fine motor, gross motor and speech and language development. The multidisciplinary nature of therapeutic yoga makes it ideal for a child with developmental delays, and the goals of all pediatric specialists can be supported through the natural integration of the yoga therapy program.

Telles and Naveen (1997) reported that motor coordination, social skills and mental ability all improved when yoga was used for rehabilitation with a mentally handicapped population.

### Exchanges/deletions

Provide support for any postures and transitions that the child has not yet mastered developmentally.

### Yoga focus for developmental delay

- Full yoga pose sequence: see Chapter Four.

- Games to build strength: see pages 146–147.

- Mudra and mantra activities: see pages 48–49.

## DOWN SYNDROME

The child diagnosed with Down syndrome receives several opportunities to build strength through maintaining a weight bearing yoga pose. The developmental nature of the yoga therapy sequence allows children with Down syndrome to move through various poses to strengthen their base of support. Arms up against gravity, weight bearing on legs and arms, nasal breathing, and practice with isolated finger movement all provide this population with ample opportunities to improve their tone, strength and dexterity.

In her book *Yoga for the Special Child*, Sonia Sumar (1998) describes the wonders of a yoga practice for, first, her own daughter and later for many other children with Down syndrome. Her background as a yoga teacher helped her support her daughter and resulted in positive changes in her daughter's development, including her school work.

The automatic opportunity to communicate with gestures is a positive feature of yoga when treating children with Down syndrome, because many use sign language or total communication (sign language and words) to express their thoughts, wants and needs. The simple vowel–consonant combination used to produce "OM" is developmentally easy for a child who is just beginning to speak. The sequenced mudras can be kept simple or made more challenging, depending on the fine motor skill of the child.

### Exchanges/deletions

Avoid rolling onto the cervical vertebrae in spinal roll pose. If the child has a history of cardiac problems, keep inversion postures of Triangle, Downward dog and Umbrella to a minimum. Rather than asking the child to close their mouth, I simply remind them to breathe through their nose.

### Yoga focus for Down syndrome

- Nasal inhalation in breathing games: see pages 152–154.

- Strength building poses: see all duration poses under the Low Tone section of this chapter see pages 171 and 177.

- Games to build strength: see pages 146—147.

- Eye exercises: eye exercises are done not by moving the head, but by moving the eyes in the direction requested. Have the child look up as high as they can by following your finger. Then have them look down as far as they can. Repeat this from side to side. It is important that just the eyes are moving and not the entire head.

## EMOTIONAL SENSITIVITY

Yoga provides an environment that encourages relaxation and centeredness. A yoga venue encourages environmental calm and the opportunity for inner reflection. In this context there is the potential to reduce anxiety and release sadness and to replace these feelings with a calm and more joyful awareness.

The experience of balance and wholeness is crucial for a child experiencing bipolar disorder. Yoga can be an excellent addition to the child's repertoire for facilitating positive feelings. The benefits of yoga for depression are reviewed in depth by Amy Weintraub in her book *Yoga for Depression* (2004), where she provides breathing and posture exercises to improve overall state of mind. Weintraub has developed a CD with breathing exercises to treat depression (Weintraub 2003).

### Exchanges/deletions

None.

### Yoga focus for emotional well-being

- Breathing games: see pages 152—154.

- Games to build confidence: see pages 148–150.

- Mudra and mantra games: see pages 147–148.

- *Savasana*: see pages 50–51.

## FLUENCY DISORDER

Research into fluency disorders, such as stuttering, has reported that modified vocal parameters (i.e., volume, rate, and rhythm of speech) can help facilitate fluency. Focused breathing activities in the yoga therapy sequence can facilitate this process, and receiving and retaining information can occur more quickly and at deeper levels when in a meditative state. In this state of balance there is potential to improve fluency of speech.

Yoga mudras sequenced to mantras provide repeated opportunities to simultaneously sing and clap to a rhythm. Movements incorporating the skill of crossing the midline of the body also support integration. Learning to follow rhythm at various rates with fine motor skills can help with the motor planning skills for finer production of speech.

In a recently published book, *Yoga for Stuttering*, J. M. Balakrishnan (2009) provides voice, breathing and physical exercises based on the ancient traditions of Nada, Hatha and Raja yoga to promote fluency of speech in individuals who have not found success with traditional methods.

## *Exchanges/deletions*

None.

## *Yoga focus for fluency*

- Breathing games: see pages 152–154.

- Mudra and mantra games: see pages 147–148.

- Musical instruments: see page 151.

- *Savasana*: see pages 50–51.

## HEMIPARESIS

I never tire of addressing the natural and automatic benefits that a yoga program offers. One of the greatest needs for a child diagnosed with hemiparesis, or weakness of one side of the body, is to be given multiple opportunities to engage in bilateral activities—activities that use both sides of the body. Yoga stimulates both sides of the body at each developmental level, from lying supine, up and through all transitions into standing. The very foundation of yoga is based on using both sides of the body, so a therapeutic yoga program like this will naturally support the needs of a child with hemiparesis.

The ordered postures in the yoga therapy sequence allow repetitive opportunities to improve motor planning. Through gross motor practice in *asana* (Sanskrit word for yoga posture) to fine motor sequences of mudras, the child's brain can be stimulated for rehabilitation. The breath work in yoga allows greater oxygenation of the constricted side of the body and the opportunity to alter brainwaves for deeper integration. Stimulating the weak side of the body can reduce the development of compensations on the stronger side of the body.

A well-balanced, energetic body gives the child a sense of wholeness and balance. Although this may not be demonstrated by the physical structure, it may be felt within the child.

### Exchanges/deletions

Observe the child during weight bearing activities and help her, if needed, in establishing the foundation for a pose (e.g., Cat, Dog, and Table).

### Yoga focus for hemiparesis

- Games using props and toys: see pages 150–151.
- Games to build strength: see pages 146–147.
- Downward dog pose: see pages 94–95.
- Cat pose: see pages 92–93.

## HIGH TONE

In general yoga has the effect of stretching and elongating the body, and so provides an excellent setting for the child with high tone and/or body constrictions. The use of focused breath triggers relaxation, and the yoga poses encourage stretch, elongation and alignment. With repeated sessions, the body moves more easily into a relaxed state, and each breath helps further elongation and/or range of movement.

Tight heel cords (Achilles tendons) can be gently stretched in the poses of Downward dog and Squat. Butterfly pose encourages improved hip flexibility towards external rotation, while Arch pose encourages flat feet on the mat. Within each pose, there is a target for improvement, and, over sessions, there is the opportunity for the body to gently change.

*Exceptions/deletions*

None.

*Yoga focus for high tone*

- Full body stretch: see pages 52–53.
- Leg extensions: see pages 54–57.
- Lying spinal twist: see pages 58–61.
- Downward dog pose: see pages 94–95.
- Volcano pose: see pages 70–73.

## LANGUAGE DELAY AND/OR DISORDER

The yoga therapy setting naturally stimulates many of the language concepts that are crucial to the development of understanding and using language. The automatic use of gesture and simple song support a total communication approach and elicit multiple levels of expression. Mirroring the poses creates support for children who first learn to communicate by imitating. Yoga is a peaceful environment for receptive language practice, as each pose is explained with simple directions. One- and two-step directions are rehearsed as a natural response to the class. Using simple chants with Hindu words not only eliminates semantic attachment to the words but also provides simple consonant–vowel/vowel–consonant combinations. "OM" is one of the earliest and easiest vowel–consonant combinations and is close to a child's earliest vocabulary of "mom" or "mama." The incorporation of mudras, or hand postures, supports children who may be communicating at a gesture level. The gross motor movements of yoga encourage motor expression and invite success for those children who are not able to communicate verbally.

Body awareness supports early language skills by providing a natural context for learning the content category of position. The child learns the concepts of *in front of*, *in back of*, *above*, *together*, and *to the side* by engaging in each direction. Quality is practiced through concepts of *soft*, *deep*, *slow* and *smooth*. Receptive language skills are stimulated when the instructor moves through the postures and demonstrates the movement for the words she is using.

### Exchanges/deletions

None.

### Yoga focus for language delay and/or disorder

- Mudra and mantra games: see pages 147–148.

- Breathing games: see pages 152–154.

- Games to build confidence: see pages 148–150.

## LOW TONE

Yoga provides an excellent opportunity for overall body toning. The body is strengthened through weight bearing poses, transitions over the base of support, and numerous opportunities to move portions of the body against gravity.

Lotus posture (sitting with legs crossed in front) facilitates a desired sitting posture for children with low tone by inhibiting w-sitting (see page 80) and encouraging the use of trunk muscles to transition in and out of sitting. The weight bearing poses of Cat, Dog and Table encourage strengthening and endurance. Butterfly breathing, Half Moon, Sway, Triangle and Volcano all require the use of arms against gravity. The movement of engaging in Helicopter and spinal roll can stimulate increased tone, and spinal roll works the abdominals for improved trunk support. The chest-expander pose and upward-facing Dog offer improved extension of the upper thoracic area of the back (which can often be underdeveloped in children with low tone). The continuous praise of straight back posture and head erect on neck remind those with low tone to align and lengthen. These are messages that are provided to all students, without singling out a child with low tone.

### Exchanges/deletions

None.

### Yoga focus for low tone

- Lotus sitting: see page 129.
- Spinal rolls (to alert tone and strengthen abdominals): see pages 64–66.
- Umbrella (see pages 112–113) and upward-facing dog (see pages 96–97) poses for upper thoracic extension.

There are many occasions when you may wish to have a child hold a pose longer than she has previously been able to in order to build strength. This is where creative intervention may be helpful. Please note how I use these activities to engage the child and encourage her to maintain a pose for longer simply by distracting the child with a creative task.

TABLE

In this pose I ask the child to explain to me what they are serving from their table. They may describe the plates, utensils, and of course the menu. This is fun, as well as helping the child develop strength and endurance.

Nutrition is often discussed during this pose, and there is an opportunity to review the benefits of healthy food. You can learn a great deal about a child by learning whether they seek carbohydrates for increased serotonin production and comfort, or whether they gravitate to tastes or textures that are highly stimulating.

ARCH

To maintain a longer Arch pose, we discuss what is passing under our bridge. We may be providing a bridge over water, with ships passing under. Opening a drawbridge is an excellent image to encourage a child to lift the Arch pose higher. Any wide variety of animals may pass under the child's arch, and of course we must maintain height until the last one passes through.

VOLCANO

In order to achieve fully extended arms, I explain to the child that the volcano will erupt when their arms go higher. To motivate greater interest in this pose we discuss what is erupting from our volcano. A wide variety of objects have erupted in my classes, ranging from butterflies and toy cars to cookies. When the child understands that their arms represent the lava spewing from a volcano, they tend to have a greater range of motion.

FLOWER

Longer balance in Flower is generally achieved by telling the child that a butterfly has landed on their petals. Describing the shape, color and size of the butterfly and flower provides a reason for the child to extend the duration of the pose.

CAT

Expressing cat-like behaviors not only maintains this pose longer, but also encourages the child to balance first on one hand and then on the other. To achieve one-handed balance we pretend to lick our paw as if we were a cat. To maintain balance on one leg we create a cat's tail by lifting the other leg up in the air. Of course our cats have two tails, so that we can balance on each leg! Mewing and hissing augment the pose for duration and creativity.

To improve the overall posture I explain that the arching cat looks like a sway-backed horse that has a curved spine. To achieve a more rounded back I describe the image of the black Halloween cat that is so popular for that holiday.

### DOG

Barking, whining and growling all encourage longer mainte-nance of Downward dog pose. Encouraging the children to lift their puppy tails encourages a higher pose.

### HEAD TO KNEE

Asking the child to kiss their knee encourages greater flexion, which can develop stronger trunk support by exercising the abdominals.

### BUTTERFLY

I frequently use rhymes to prolong the butterfly pose. I will recite one line and then, utilizing closure, I let the child fill in the last word of the second line. An example of this exercise is:

"Butterfly, butterfly flies so high—

Butterfly, butterfly in the—."

The child completes the verse with "sky." This is a popular activity, and the children frequently request this game.

A second activity that I use to prolong Butterfly is to have the butterfly leave on a small adventure, and I then describe everything the butterfly sees. The children become engrossed in the story and continue to flap their wings as the butterfly travels from one spot to the next.

SPINAL TWIST

Prolonging a spinal twist is as easy as asking a child to describe what is behind them. Of course, this is not fun without imagination, and the child is encouraged to create whatever they wish. Often a story has unfolded by the time they twist in the second direction.

CHILD'S POSE

I ask the child to feel like an ice cube in this pose. To achieve a longer and more relaxed pose I explain that their arms, feet and head have melted and their body is an ice cube. I then describe them melting, which generally results in a more relaxed posture and greater benefit in this pose.

HELICOPTER

There is rarely a time that I need to encourage this pose to be longer. The children love it, and as they continue to swing, the body becomes more relaxed and the pose improves. This pose was taught to me by Sam Dworkis in a workshop specializing in restorative yoga. He encouraged each of us to prolong this pose for ten minutes, and I felt progressively better as I twisted.

TRIANGLE

I ask the child to describe where they see triangle shapes in my pose. This prolongs the pose and gives them an opportunity to describe body positions.

HALF MOON

In this pose I encourage the children to reach as high as possible. I encourage them to catch a cloud, and I frequently see not only a longer pose but a higher reach.

TREE

I have had great success with Tree pose by asking the child to stay in the pose and envision roots growing from the soles of their feet into the earth. I ask the child to see the roots grow to the center of the earth and wrap around the axis. I then ask the child to grow tall, with branches reaching toward the sky. Helping the child create a picture of the pose in greater detail extends the duration of the pose.

## POST-TRAUMATIC STRESS DISORDER (PTSD)

This diagnosis has had increased coverage as parts of our world are at war. Post-traumatic stress disorder is known as the condition that develops in soldiers who have been in battle and seen the ramifications of dying. The truth about PTSD is that it can occur in any context where an individual experiences a threat of dying. Many of our children with special needs have experienced life-threatening medical complications, and this creates fear.

Treatments that have been found helpful in the treatment of PTSD are those that facilitate calm and balance without referring to or reviewing the original trauma. Gerbarg and Brown (2005) report that, following Hurricane Katrina in September 2005, child evacuees felt less tense and aggressive by the third day of a yogic breathing program offered at the Austin Convention Center. Further benefits cited from the breathing program were improvements in the children's sleep and energy levels.

Noah Shachtman (2008) reports that the US Army is offering yoga as one of the treatment choices for soldiers returning home from Iraq and Afghanistan with PTSD, and that the US government is funding research for alternative means to treat PTSD, as well as traumatic brain injury.

## Exchanges/deletions

None.

## Yoga focus for PTSD

- Breathing games: see pages 152–154.

- *Savasana*: see pages 50–51.

- Mudra and mantra games: see pages 147–148.

- Games to build confidence: see pages 148–150.

## SENSORY INTEGRATION DISORDER

Yoga has had positive results with children with sensory integration disorder. The three systems that are affected in a sensory integration disorder are the tactile, vestibular and proprioceptive systems. All three of these systems are impacted in the yoga program outlined in this book, and a variety of symptoms can be treated. The symptoms that can be present in sensory integration disorder—speech delay, hyperactivity, low tone, high tone, low activity, motor planning problems, tactile issues, lack of body awareness and difficulty with attention, to name a few—are all treatable through a yoga practice.

Movement is necessary to treat the vestibular system, and yoga provides opportunities with spinal rolls and Helicopter pose. Coordinated fine motor sequences are part of the battery that is used to assess Sensory Integration disorder.

Nicole Cuomo, in *Integrated Yoga. Yoga with a Sensory Integrative Approach* (2007), supports the use of yoga with children who are diagnosed with sensory integration disorder. She recommends yoga as an "enhancement to treatment."

*Exchanges/deletions*

None.

*Yoga focus for sensory integration disorder*

- Mudra and mantra games: see pages 147–148.

- Spinal rolls: see pages 64–65.

- Helicopter pose: see pages 104–105.

- Eye bag and blanket: see page 26.

- Breathing games: see pages 152–154.

## SOCIAL COMMUNICATION DELAY

Many of the skills practiced in social groups are used in a yoga session. The first step of the yoga therapy sequence requires all participants to acknowledge one another through *namasté*. This exchange promises respect and requires eye contact—two behaviors that elicit more effective communication. The context of the entire session is one of honoring one another while being responsible for your own body within the space of your yoga mat. This sets appropriate parameters of body space, as well as a tone of respect for communicating with other people.

Turn-taking is critical in communication, as one person listens while another speaks. Practicing the role of teacher in yoga allows this type of skill building: when we teach we are speaking, and, when we are not in the teaching role, we listen.

Breathing begins the session and takes the children into a relaxed state that improves focus, reduces anxiety and supports a balanced state of being. These factors create a context in which a person can communicate more easily. The heart-opening exercises are designed to open each child's heart more deeply, and this helps create more loving communications.

*Exchanges/deletions*

   None.


*Yoga focus for social communication delay*

   • Breathing games: see pages 152–154.

   • Games to develop imagination: see pages 154–156.

   • Games to build confidence: see pages 148–150.

   • Mudra and mantra games: see pages 147–148.


## SCOLIOSIS

Yoga has been found to lessen the symptoms of scoliosis. Yoga gently moves the spine through all planes of movement by elongating, rotating and bending. Yoga can stretch muscles where asymmetrical constriction exists and provide greater symmetry, reducing compensatory patterns. Structural changes that have developed over time will require gentle yoga sequences to encourage stretching, elongation and rotation.

Elise Browning Miller modified her personal scoliosis pain by practicing yoga, and now offers consultations and conducts workshops to help others. In her book *Yoga for Scoliosis* (updated in 2007) she recommends various poses to relax the muscles, lengthen the spine and experience the healing effects of *savasana*.


*Exchanges/deletions*

   None.


*Yoga focus for scoliosis*

   • Full body stretch with breathing: see pages 52–53.

   • Cat pose: see pages 92–93.

- Triangle pose: see pages 114–117.

- Supine spinal twist: see pages 58–61.

- Sitting spinal twist: see pages 84–87.

- Helicopter pose: see pages 104–105.

# 8

## THE RESPONSE: YOGIS AND PARENTS

This final chapter of this book is devoted to children and their parents and their statements of how yoga therapy has changed their lives. These children have been practicing the yoga program on a weekly schedule over a period of months to years. They are the true stars of yoga therapy.

### JOEY

"I feel relaxed when I come in the yoga room and when I am done I feel more relaxed and great. I can breathe relaxed and soft. Yoga lets all the stress out of me, like one day I was so stressed with school and my work unfinished and after yoga it didn't bother me."

## Joey's mother, Tina

"Our nine-year-old son, Joey, was diagnosed with a liver disease called Alagille's syndrome in early infancy. It is a very rare, multi-symptomatic disorder that is characterized by a reduced number of small bile ducts within the liver combined with abnormalities in other organs, including the heart, eyes, spine, kidneys, lungs, and pancreas. From early infancy, Joey's complex medical condition has caused substantial developmental delays and has required close medical monitoring and intervention.

Due to our son's medical condition, he has required a great deal of therapy since birth. His obvious developmental delays were addressed through traditional therapy methods, including physical therapy, speech therapy, and occupational therapy. All of these therapies were invaluable; however, there were still some quality of life issues that were not being addressed. We realized that there were pieces to the puzzle missing, that could potentially improve our son's health and overall well-being.

Therapeutic yoga is one of these puzzle pieces that has greatly improved our son's life. We began therapeutic yoga as a suggested therapy to help Joey with his balance and motor skills, as well as a means to help relieve the stiffness of body that he suffers due to his illness. All of these issues are certainly addressed by his yoga sessions. We quickly discovered, however, that yoga is a discipline that has many more benefits that we did not expect.

The illness and physical discomfort that our son has suffered his entire life, coupled with his developmental delays, have caused Joey to be detached from his own body. His poor motor planning and his inability to recognize his own physical discomfort were limiting his activities. Yoga has been instrumental in helping him to better connect with his own body. His balance and motor planning have improved, resulting in less falling and injuries. He has also shown a great deal of improvement in recognizing how his body is feeling and communicating those feelings. Prior to yoga, it was very rare that Joey told us anything about how he was physically feeling, whether it was good or bad.

Joey has always had a great deal of sensory issues that have made his life more difficult and required a great deal of therapy. Our experience with yoga showed that it also was extremely useful in addressing his sensory problems. The mind—body connection that yoga fosters helped in addressing his oversensitivity to the world around him, including sound, sights, tastes, and textures.

The quiet and calm of yoga have also been extremely beneficial for our son. He has been diagnosed as ADHD, and he is a very physically active child. Along with his ADHD he occasionally has episodes of anxiety and obsessive worrying. His life is also extremely scheduled and very busy with school, therapy and doctor's appointments. Yoga is a safe and quiet place that relieves his anxiety and raises his spirits. He has gained valuable skills in self-calming and can even practice his yoga at home.

Lastly, the basic philosophy of yoga that unites the mind, body and spirit is a philosophy that we have come to see as invaluable for our son. Yoga has allowed him to be successful at a physical endeavor, on his own terms. It has increased his self-esteem and taught him to think about the value of his own body and health. As he continues to face physical challenges brought on by his medical condition, yoga can be a healthy outlet. He may not always be able to control some aspects of his life affected by his illness; however, when he practices yoga he can have control over his body, mind, and spirit to strengthen his self-esteem and sense of well being."

## ZACHARY

"I can tell I am doing better with yoga because I can think better. Whenever I think about something I know the answer better. Yoga helps me get rid of sadness. I feel positive inside instead of negative. I feel good about helping teach the class.

Before yoga class, I have come from school, and I feel like my brain is tired. After yoga my emotions calm down and my body feels relaxed but also energized. My brain thinks better again."

### Zachary's mother, Wendy

"When my case manager suggested yoga about five years ago, I kind of just laughed and thought, with Zachary's lack of motor planning and flexibility he would never be able to do yoga. Now every time someone mentions yoga I have many accomplishments to share from Zachary's experience with yoga. He can calm himself when anxiety and nervousness sets in by using the breathing techniques he learned in yoga. I just need to give him a little reminder to do yoga breathing. He breathes much deeper and slower and this calms him.

"His speech has also come a long way. I can see Zachary concentrating while doing yoga poses, and I see this same concentration when he is thinking about what he wants to say. He is able to put his thoughts together into sequence so whatever he is saying makes sense. His speech has improved in yoga more intensely than when he studied with a speech therapist. He gets to communicate with others in the group yoga setting and share his ideas. Then there is the relaxing that comes from the deep, slow breathing, and he sleeps much better and sounder at night.

"In the therapeutic yoga group, each child teaches different poses to the others in the group. This has really boosted Zachary's confidence. You can see improved confidence in school when he has to answer questions in class or do oral reports.

"I have seen very positive changes in Zachary from the yoga, and I would recommend it to anyone."

## MATTHEW

"After I do yoga I feel more open, exercised, relaxed and calm. Yoga also makes me more limber and makes me feel more in tune with myself. I have noticed that my habit of 'happy hands' is less when I have done yoga."

*Matthew's mother, Karen*

"Matthew has benefited greatly from yoga, especially in his ability to calm himself. He has also gained more flexibility in his very tight joints. Motor planning has improved since he started yoga. He is more in touch with his feelings as well as his severe sensory issues.

"Now that I have seen what yoga has done for Matthew I try to incorporate more yoga into their daily lives. I also try to do more yoga myself!"

## JONATHAN

"Yoga makes me feel good, more like a pretzel. I like yoga because it is fun because we play games."

*Jonathan's mother, Karen*

"I believe Jonathan has benefited from yoga by demonstrating more strength and body awareness. He is more aware of the breath and is able to control his breath much better. His respiratory system seems stronger to me, too. I feel that yoga has made an impact on my life by giving me more awareness on a multidimensional level, all levels working together."

## BRITTANY

"I like yoga."

*Brittany's father*

"I have seen that Brittany now can go to bed by herself. Before she started yoga she wanted her mother to lie down with her and it took a long time to get her to go to sleep. Now, she goes to bed all on her own and is able to go to sleep right away and sleeps much better.

"We also see that Brittany is able to stop making the strange sounds that autistic children can make. When we are riding in the car sometimes Brittany starts making screeching sounds that are very difficult to listen to. When we tell her to do her yoga she starts breathing and stops the sounds. After doing the breathing she does not make the sounds again."

## Brittany's mother

"After yoga Brittany started using longer and more difficult words. She was able to say 'computador' when she wanted to play on the computer. She also began using two words together a lot of the time, and before she had mostly used one word, and only sometimes two words together.

"Brittany also understands stories much better when we read to her. Since she has been taking yoga she is easier going."

## CHASE

"Yoga helps me concentrate. I also can be quieter, and when I breathe deep, I can balance better. After a yoga class I feel really good and also after the guided story.

"When I come to yoga class I feel like I'm going to have an exciting day and at the end of class I am happy that I was there. I feel peaceful in my body and I know that I will be peaceful for the day. I can think clear because I don't have all the things coming up in my mind and I don't have to think all these things at once.

"Yoga makes me feel calm and that I don't have to worry. It teaches me like when I'm mad I can breathe and I don't have to worry about it any more. I won't go over and argue with someone. I'll calm myself down, forget about it, and I won't have to worry about it."

## Chase's mother, Cori

"Chase has a diagnosis of autism and Attention Deficit Hyperactivity Disorder. He is nine years old and has been in yoga for four years.

"As a parent I have been greatly impressed with the progress Chase has made while participating in therapeutic yoga. Often he arrives at class in a little body that is filled with stress and stiffness and emerges following his yoga time so content, calm and whole. It continues to amaze me!

"I am appreciative that Nancy has given him skills that he can use outside the yoga 'classroom.' Calm, deep breathing (although just one part of yoga) is a technique that has helped Chase at school, with peers, at soccer, even while waiting in a long line! I anticipate that therapeutic yoga will continue to bless Chase's life well into adulthood."

## MIA

"I like yoga. Yoga makes me happy and yoga is fun."

## Mia's mother, Cathy

"My daughter, Mia, has Down syndrome and has been participating in therapeutic yoga for the past two and a half years. Mia sees many different therapists such as speech, physical therapy, and occupational therapy, but yoga is a time for Mia to relax and be introspective. It builds her confidence and is a special activity for her to enjoy. I feel that yoga helps her in many areas of development: strengthening weak muscles, working on breath and speech through poses, songs, and chants, fine motor with chimes and other poses, intellectually with concentration and focus. To me therapeutic yoga addresses many of the challenges that Mia has to work on in a fun and positive way."

## AMY

"Yoga makes me feel good, happy. I also eat better and I talk better."

### Amy's mother, Theresa

"Amy is my 13-year-old daughter who was diagnosed at 18-months-old with global developmental delays. She also received diagnosis for cerebral palsy, apraxia of speech, and falls somewhere in the autism spectrum.

"We started the standard therapies—speech, occupational therapy and physical therapy. There were also some not so traditional therapies we did, such as swim therapy, therapeutic horseback riding and yoga. We were introduced to yoga to assist Amy in improving her speech, learning to relax and to not be so anxious, to develop more tone in her neck muscles, to improve her sleep and help her sleep through the night and to give her a break from traditional therapy. Yoga was fun and different. Amy started yoga at age five; she has very low muscle tone and had a very small vocabulary of words. She used basic sign language and was using an augmentative communication device.

"The first year I wasn't sure what we were getting from yoga, but felt we needed to stay with it because we were seeing some increase in her speech. She also started working in a group and was getting some social skills interaction with other kids like her. Over time we saw that she was able to relax and get in her yoga mind frame and calm herself down. For example, a trip to the dentist was something that was not easy for Amy or the staff that tried to examine and treat her. Any work that needed to be done, she needed sedation. We recently went for a check-up and I could tell she was starting to have a breakdown. I told her to close her eyes and think about yoga. She immediately closed her eyes and started to chant/hum and her hands were in her OM position, and she opened her mouth and the dentist went to work cleaning and examining her teeth.

"I was so very happy that we had put the time and effort into yoga because for her to self-regulate her behavior and relax was truly amazing. Yoga will always be a part of Amy's life and routine and the friendships she has found in yoga will also be lasting."

## NICKY

"Yoga drowns out stress or worries, and it fills your head with positive thoughts. Yoga also gives me hope for something you want to come true. It makes you feel hopeful about those dreams coming true, especially if I help to make that happen.

"After yoga class I feel happy and calm. I don't know how, but it makes me feel better about myself."

### Nicky's mother, Ana

"Nicky has been participating in yoga for one-and-a-half years. We think yoga is a very helpful therapy for him. Yoga helps Nicky to learn; to relax, to breathe, to reduce anxiety, to regulate his sensory issues and self-control. It makes him feel comfortable and accepted in a friendly, positive and safe environment.

"This opportunity helps Nicky and the other kids to develop physical confidence and understand their bodies. Yoga balances the limited physical activities and opportunities offered at school.

"Yoga is a complete therapy that helps him not only with the postures for his gross motor skill and coordination, but also to belong to a social group, to gain confidence and nourishment for his soul."

## CLAIRE

"Yoga teaches me lessons about life and what I can do. I have learned you worry only about how I am doing in yoga and not what other people are doing, like paying attention or not. Yoga calms me down and I think the meditation stories are especially relaxing. Yoga helps me get my mind off of bad or embarrassing things that happen during the day.

"Yoga helps me understand who I am and why we are around. I have learned you are more than just your face, your hair and your body. I am life."

## LIA

"Yoga is refreshing. It makes me feel like I have taken a bath except instead of just my body feeling clean, my soul is too! Sometimes before I do yoga I do not want to go because I am upset from being made fun of at school. After yoga I feel a lot better and I am glad I did it. It makes me feel ready to get on with my day and much calmer."

### Lia and Claire's mother, Carol

"My two daughters, Lia (12) and Claire (9) both have been diagnosed with high functioning autism and they have both benefited so much from their yoga sessions. Lia has a very bright and busy mind and we have found that yoga has helped calm her thinking. After taking a short break from yoga several years ago, Lia seemed to be having a harder time controlling her anxiety and behavior. This especially was happening at school, which can be a challenging and stressful place for her. When we asked her what she thought might help her feel better she requested to return to yoga which she stated 'helped calm me down.' The breathing, mind—body connection awareness, and creative imagery used in Nancy's yoga sessions help Lia focus and channel all of her wonderful mind energy. It seems to soothe and calm her, and you can see the difference in her face as soon as she comes out of a session. We have seen a lot of improvement in her ability to calm herself at school and at home."

"Claire is also a very bright girl, but her language skills are more delayed by her autism. Yoga has helped Claire's speech with breath control and oral motor strength. She loves to do poses, and yoga also works to help focus and calm her thinking. Claire gets in a calm state and is able to create and say wonderful meditations stories with her friends, which she says 'helps her think of this better' and that yoga helps 'people make more sense' to her. We've also seen great improvement in her coordination and sense of rhythm."

## KATY

"Yoga has helped me be calm. I don't get as angry as I used to. I am able to be more flexible and I can reach farther and keep my balance. Like when I was in my bed and I wanted to reach for a blanket that was farther away from my bed. I reached out and was able to get the blanket and keep my balance without falling out of my bed. Also when a boy dropped his pencil in class I was able to bend and reach from my desk to pick it up. I was surprised I could reach that far without falling."

### Katy's mother, Laura

"Katy has been taking yoga instruction for a year now and had initially started off in a small group session. Right away she enjoyed going to yoga class. She would love to tell us about the new things she learned. I noticed that she really felt excitement on the days we were coming to yoga. She does not express a lot of interest in areas outside of her computer or playstation, so we are constantly looking for other activities to involve her in.

"Katy has a medical diagnosis of autism, although she is considered very high functioning. She has always had a moderately high level of anxiety and some compulsive type behaviors as well.

"Probably the biggest change we saw in Katy came when we switched her from a small group class to a one-on-one session. It was right at the time that puberty hit and things at school began to fall apart. Her grades were slipping and several of her friendships fell apart. She is in the 7th grade, and it has been a very rough year for her.

"When I pick her up after school she is almost always tense and very shut down. On Wednesdays she has her yoga session and we usually arrive with her in a pretty bad mood. She tells me on the drive over that she just wants to stay at home in her room and not go anywhere, a sure sign of how much anxiety she carries around with her. After her yoga session she always emerges like a new kid! She is talkative and bubbly on the drive home, and Wednesday night typically tends to be our best school night of the week. She is easier to work with on homework and I've noticed she is more helpful around the house, offering to help set the table or even just initiate conversation with me as I'm preparing dinner.

"One thing she has started doing at night is to listen to music in her room. It has a calming effect on her and I think it is her attempt to emulate the calmness she feels at your studio. She notices the quiet and peaceful feeling in your space and associates it with feeling good. I know she is able to talk during her sessions and I believe that has really helped her to be able to relieve some of her school stress, so she leaves yoga with both her mind and body feeling better.

"I think yoga is extremely beneficial to Katy and I hope that it will be something she can continue to do into her adult years as a way to help her manage her anxiety. I see that it helps her feel more in control of herself and has a very positive effect on her behavior and attitude."

## VALERIE

"Yoga makes me feel better. I like Butterfly and Flower pose. I feel happier after I do yoga."

## ROBERT

"Yoga makes me feel better and at ease. Yoga helps me get through the day and the next day. It has helped me become a more relaxed person. I am more able to breathe in joy, calm, and peace, and it brings happier thoughts."

### *Valerie and Robert's mother, Irma*

"I would like to talk to you about both of my kids—Valerie, who was diagnosed with high functioning autism with movement disorder and Robert who was diagnosed Tourette's syndrome and hyperactivity.

"Yoga has been a key to Val's ability to see herself as a person, with different perspectives. To see this transition is heartwarming to witness. One of the most interesting experiences is to watch Valerie look at our photo albums and recall with amazing detail those event experiences. She talks with such emotion of both excitement and distress at times, like she is wondering what happened with the time. She asks what has happened to the particular clothes she was wearing in different photos or where a particular picture was taken.

"We have been able to see our daughter blossom into a young lady, able to carry on a conversation about her day and her activities. Yoga has had a significant and positive impact on Valerie's life as well as the whole family's.

"Robert has also received great benefit from his participation in yoga. The biggest change we have seen in our son is his ability to see the world around him and how he fits into it. Robert has also gained more awareness of self and his personal space and the importance of respecting the space of others.

"In short, both of our children have derived untold benefits from their participation in yoga and we would recommend it to any as a viable treatment for many special needs children."

## SALICIA'S MOTHER, TANYA

"Salicia is three years old and diagnosed with hypotonic cerebral palsy and sensory integration disorder. Salicia has been in yoga therapy for five weeks and is showing us Downward dog pose at home. I am hearing more words, sometimes two new words a day, and she is combining two words together. Before we started yoga she used very few words. She is imitating many things that I say. Yesterday she said 'popcorn' and 'clock' for the very first time. She loves to sing songs and claps to the singing."

## RUSSEL

"Yoga helped me walk without a cane and helps me balance. When I started yoga I could not get down on the mat without Nancy helping me, now I do it all by myself. My arm is stronger and I use it better now."

### Russel's mother, Lisa

"Yoga was our last chance for Russel. He suffered a stroke and required therapy for all of his developmental areas including speech, occupational, and physical therapy. When three months had passed the therapists discharged Russel and explained they could do no more for him. It was when we started yoga that Russel began to show improvement. He was able to support himself better in walking, move up and down from the floor by himself, and his speech improved. If we had not had yoga there might not have been any further improvement from Russel."

# REFERENCES

Balakrishnan, J. M. (2009) *Yoga for Stuttering: Unifying the Voice, Breath, Mind and Body to Achieve Fluent Speech*. Berkeley: North Atlantic Books.

Betts, D. E. and Betts, S. W. (2006) *Yoga for Children with Autism Spectrum Disorders: A Step-by-Step Guide for Parents and Caregivers*. London: Jessica Kingsley Publishers.

Bobath, K. (1980) *A Neurophysiological Basis for the Treatment of Cerebral Palsy (Clinics in Developmental Medicine)*. Lavenham: The Lavenham Press.

Cooper, S., Osborne, J., Newton, S., Harrison, V., Thompson, Coon, J., Lewis, S. and Tattersfield, A. (2003) "The effect of two breathing exercises (Buteyko and pranayama) in asthma: a randomized controlled trial." *Thorax 58*, 8, 674–9.

Cuomo, N. (2007) *Integrated Yoga. Yoga with a Sensory Integrative Approach*. London: Jessica Kingsley Publishers.

Dworkis, S. (1997) *Recovery Yoga: a Practical Guide for Chronically Ill, Injured, and Post-operative People*. New York: Three Rivers Press.

Gerbarg, P. L. and Brown, R. P. (2005) "Yoga: a breath of relief for Hurricane Katrina refugees." *Current Psychiatry Online, 4*, 10, 55–67.

Haffner, J., Roos, J., Goldstein, N., Parger, P. and Resch, F. (2006) 'The effectiveness of body-oriented methods of therapy in the treatment of attention-deficit hyperactivity disorder (ADHD): results of a controlled pilot study'. *Zeitschrift für Kinder und Jugendpsychiatrie und Psychotherapie 34*, 1, 37–47.

Jayasinghe, S. R. (2004) "Yoga in cardiac health (a review.)" *European Journal of Cardiovascular Prevention and Rehabilitation, 11*, 369–375.

Kriyananda, G. (1976) "The Spiritual Science of Kriya Yoga." Chicago: The Temple of Kriya Yoga.

Miller, E. B. (2007) "Yoga for Scoliosis with Elise Browning Miller: Therapeutic Back Care. Reduce Pain and Improve Posture." Innerselfmarket, available at www.yogaforscoliosis.com, accessed 24 October 2009.

Oken, B. S. (2004) "Randomized control trial of yoga and exercise in multiple sclerosis." *Neurology 62*, 2058–2064.

Shachtman, N. (2008) "Army's New PTSD Treatments: Yoga, Reiki, 'Bioenergy'." Danger Room. Accessed 5/1/2009 at www.wired.com/dangerroom/2008/03/army-bioenergy/

Seattle Children's Hospital, Seattle Cancer Care Alliance Inpatient Care Unit "Our Services." www.seattlechildrens.org/clinics-programs/scca/

Sumar, S. (1998) *Yoga for the Special Child. A Therapeutic Approach for Infants and Children with Down Syndrome, Cerebral Palsy and Learning Disabilities.* Virginia: Special Yoga Publications.

Telles, S. and Naveen, K. V. (1997) "Yoga for rehabilitation: an overview." *Indian Journal of Medical Sciences 51*, 4, 123–7.

Weintraub, A. (2003) *Breathe to Beat the Blues: Manage your Mood with your Breath.* Tuscon, AZ: Yoga to Beat the Blues Productions, available to order from www.yogafordepression.com.

Weintraub, A. (2004) *Yoga for Depression. A Compassionate Guide to Relieve Suffering Through Yoga.* New York: Broadway Books.

Williams, N. (2000) *Songs to Grow On. A Children's Yoga Program CD.* Tuscon, AZ: The Garden House, available to www.yogatherapy4kids.com

# Resources

## BOOKS

*Anatomy of Movement.* Blandine Calais-Germain (1993). Eastland Press.

*Anatomy of the Spirit.* Caroline Myss (1996). Crown Publishing.

*Breathe: Yoga for Teens.* Mary Kaye Chryssicas (2007). DK Publishing.

*Integrated Yoga.* Nicole Cuomo (2007). Jessica Kingsley Publishers.

*Recovery Yoga. A Practical Guide for Chronically Ill, Injured, and Post-Operative People.* Sam Dworkis (1997). Three Rivers Press.

*The Breathing Book. Good Health and Vitality Through Essential Breath Work.* Donna Farhi (1996). Henry Holt and Co.

*The Spiritual Science of Kriya Yoga.* Goswami Kriyananda (first edition 1976, fifth edition 1998). Published by the Temple of Kriya Yoga.

*The Treasure in Your Heart. Stories and Yoga for Peaceful Children.* Sydney Solis (2007). The Mythic Yoga Studio.

*Yoga Calm for Children.* Lynea and James Gillen (2007). Three Pebbles Press.

*Yoga for Children with Autism Spectrum Disorders. A Step-by-Step Guide for Parents and Caregivers.* Dion E. and Stacey W. Betts (2006). Jessica Kingsley Publishers.

*Yoga for Children. Simple Movements and Games You and Your Kids can do Together to Help them Grow Strong and Flexible.* Mary Stewart and Kathy Phillips (1992). Simon & Schuster.

*Yoga for Depression. A Compassionate Guide to Relieve Suffering Through Yoga.* Amy Weintraub (2004). Broadway Books.

*Yoga for the Special Child. A Therapeutic Approach for Infants and Children with Down Syndrome, Cerebral Palsy and Learning Disabilities.* Sonia Sumar (1998). Special Yoga Publications.

## JOURNALS

*Australian Yoga Life.* www.ayl.com.au/

*Fit Yoga.* www.fityoga.com

*The Yoga Journal.* www.yogajournal.com

*Yoga 4 Everybody.* www.yoga4everybody.com

*Yoga and Health.* www.yogaandhealthmag.co.uk/

*Yoga Magazine.* www.yogamagazine.co.uk/

*Yogi Times.* www.yogitimes.com

*Yoga + Joyful Living.* www.himalayaninstitute.org/yogaplus/index.aspx

*International Journal of Yoga Therapy.* www.iayt.org/site/publications/journal.php

*Yoga Magazine.* www.yogamag.net/subs.shtml

## CHILDREN'S YOGA SITES

*All for Kids.* www.all4kidsuk.com

*Radiant Child Yoga.* www.childrensyoga.com

*Yoga Calm for Children.* www.yogacalm.org

*Yoga for the Special Child.* www.specialyoga.com

*Yoga 4 Kids.* www.yogatherapy4kids.com

## YOGA ASSOCIATIONS

International Association of Yoga Therapists. www.iayt.org/publications/ytip/sep05.htm

International Yoga Teacher's Association. www.iyta.org.au

Atlantic Canada's Yoga Teachers Association. www.yogaatlantic.ca/

British Yoga Teachers' Association. www.britishyogateachersassociation.org.uk

Yoga Teachers' Association of Australia. www.tasker.yogateachers.asn.au

Yoga Alliance. www.yogaalliance.org

# GLOSSARY

**Anatomy:** study of the physical body structure.

**Apraxia:** inconsistent ability to motor plan speech.

**Bilateral:** any activity that involves the use of both sides of the body. For example, clapping is a bilateral activity.

**Chakra:** an energy center located in the invisible, energetic body.

**Directionality:** the faculty of knowing in which direction your body, or parts of your body, are moving.

**Extension:** a lengthening and opening of the body at one or more joints.

**Flexion:** a folding in and bending of the body at one or more joints.

**Graded:** of quality. A graded movement is accomplished with a high skill of balance.

**Guided imagery:** narration of a positive story or experience to the child or group as they rest with eyes closed.

**Hatha:** "Hatha" is the combination of two different Sanskrit words. *Ha* and *tha* mean "the breath of the sun" and "the breath of the moon," respectively.

**Hemiparesis:** one-sided weakness in the body.

**Inversion:** any yoga pose that requires at least the head and upper body to be upside-down. A headstand is a total inversion.

**Lateral:** of or to the side.

**Mantra:** a Sanskrit term for a sacred chant.

**Motor planning:** a sequenced series of movements that completes a given task.

**Mudra:** sacred hand postures used in the practice of yoga.

**Multidimensional:** involving more than one dimension in any given situation.

**Multidisciplinary:** involving more than one discipline or area of focus, i.e. an activity that stimulates both fine and gross motor skills.

*Namasté*: a greeting in Sanskrit meaning "I honor the light in you."

**Natural setting:** any setting that a child would normally include in his or her activities of daily living.

**Neuro-Developmental Treatment:** a therapy treatment developed by Berta and Karl Bobath in the treatment of children diagnosed with cerebral palsy.

**OM:** the original sound of creation. A Sanskrit mantra.

**Physiology:** the study of the movement of the body.

**Pincer grasp:** holding an object by pinching the thumb and index finger together.

**Positive affirmations:** declarations made about one's self in a positive state.

**Proprioception:** a "sixth sense" or faculty whereby stimuli from skin, muscles, joints, and tendons are fed back to the brain via the nervous system and generate "body image" and body awareness.

**Reiki:** an energy treatment involving transference of universal life force as the practitioner positions his hands at a slight distance from the surface of the body.

*Savasana:* a Sanskrit term meaning "total relaxation."

**Scoliosis:** an abnormal curvature in the spine.

*Shanti:* the Sanskrit word meaning "peace."

**Solar plexus:** the area of the body located above the navel and below the ribcage.

**Tactile:** involving touch.

**Vestibular system:** the organs of balance located in the inner ear; part of the sensory system that enables the body to sustain balance and orientation as it moves through space.

**Yoga:** Sanskrit word meaning "union," including the union of physical structure and subtle energy.